Presented to Vashti D. Garwood
By Mrs James Woodmansee
Urbana O.
June 1. 1894.

THE

CLOSING SCENE:

A VISION.

In Twelve Books.

BY JAMES WOODMANSEE.

Like the baseless fabric of a Vision,—
The cloud-capp'd Towers, the gorgeous Palaces,
The solemn Temples, the great Globe itself,
Yea, all which it inherit shall dissolve,
And like this insubstantial pageant faded—
Leave not a rack behind!—SHAKSPEARE.

Cincinnati:
PRINTED AT THE METHODIST BOOK CONCERN,
FOR THE AUTHOR.

R. P. THOMPSON, PRINTER.
1857.

TO

My Very Dear Mother,

RACHEL WOODMANSEE,

WHO HATH MADE ME ALL I AM,

The Closing Scene

IS

DEDICATED

BY

HER SON,

THE

AUTHOR.

Let me alone——I go
To a land of darkness, as Darkness itself,
To the Shadow of Death without order,
Where Light, is as—Darkness!

JOB.

BOOK I.

The Closing Scene.

BOOK I.

FIRST Cause of every cause—Almighty Cause!
Forever present, always Ancient One,—
The life of all, great Being's dawn and end—
All-making Lord—the All in All and Sire,
From everlasting to e'erlasting—God!
Incomprehensible and infinite—
The fullness of Immensity for aye!
To whom, the Heaven of Heavens is but a seat,
A footstool Earth, and Hell—a spark of fire!

Of Thee, bereft, how dumb is every joy!
All life how dead, and worlds unnumber'd—nought!

Or speck of dust 'mid Chaos' deep profound,
A mote on bosom of Nonentity—
Too small a fiber for the scales of Nought!
And Man—(immortal image of his Sire,)
A grain of sand on vast Atlantic-wave!
Life-bubble toss'd by Being's rapid tide
To wreck on ocean of Calamity!
Atom in chamber of Infinity!
A fleeting shade on shoreless deep of Space!
A shadow-spectre in the night of Time,—
Eternal Torment's never-dying worm
On sulphurous surge in tempest-tossing Hell!

Thro' Love-divine and boundless Mercy, what?
A saint, an angel, seraph and a god
Eternal as—Thyself! When Man rebell'd,
Had sinn'd and stray'd with Vice to wretchedness
As far as Hell,—at war with God and fast
To Satan wed,—ruined, lost, and almost damn'd—
Incapable to purchase with his all
Redemption,—wishing not to be redeemed!
Wondrous in mercy, Thou in mercy gave
Thy Son—our ADVOCATE—EMMANUEL!

And—infinite of love! Man, with Thyself,
And Earth with Heaven redeem'd in their despite!
From mites of wrath, exalted men to gods!
For endless death, us life eternal gave!
For flames of Hell—home blissful in the Heavens!
Number'd with saints instead of demons damn'd,
And Mercy smiled to smile forever-more!

O! how shall Man love, venerate, adore
Thee as he ought Almighty? How for Thy
Love infinite? amazing mercy how?
For full atonement made—accession free
Thro' suffering Savior's blood on Calvary shed
Poor Fallen Nature's fell death-wound to heal?
Restoring Earth so near to God and Heaven
That rapture-breathing Prayer, spirit-soaring flies
To audience-chamber of Emmanuel,
And mingling with day-glories 'round the throne
Celestial blessings feast Contrition's heart
Melting at presence near of Deity!
And—Faith! with Heaven-besieging eye full-fix'd,
Sun-bright beholds the great Eternal there—

Full-noon of glory burning infinite—
Light, life and heaven of all the Heaven of
Heavens!

O, rise my soul! with holy Rapture rise
To adoration mute, astonishment;
With sacred awe and spirit-trembling breathe
Thy thoughts too hallow'd all for utterance,
In deep, dead-silence dumb with reverence
His name eternal musing—lost in Him!
This world from thine immortal pinions shake,
Shake imperfection—mix with Purities
Whose every thought 's a prayer and breath a
psalm,
And God their all in all eternally.

O! lean my weakness on Omnipotence,
My ignorance on Wisdom perfect lean
And imperfections all on spotless Purity:—
O! wake Thou good desires, unhallow'd chase,
And sanctify this luke-warm heart—Almighty!
Thy will to do with humbleness and love,—
O, guide an atom 'mid Creation's dust!

My being be an end, my all in all—
Supporter, father, friend,—deliverer
In danger, guide to every duty, shield
From troubles all,—my rock, defence and tow'r
Of strength thro' life, thro' death—eternity
Of endless blessedness in loving Heaven.

Spirit of God! thou—Light Ineffable!
Brood o'er the dark of my chaotic mind
As "o'er the water's face" when Nature's self
Confusion lay the bosom of Old Night:—
With Glory's flame and Thy divinity
Illume me as Thou did'st Creation then
That rose complete to magnify Thy pow'r—
Stupendous wonder grand to Angel-eye,
To mortal sight another Deity!
And me inspire the hallow'd mount sublime
Of Holy Song to soar, and tread at will
Her loftiest heights, familiar and at home.
Me, judgment give and wide expanse of thought,
Give wisdom, spirit—flaming Harp of fire
Strung with immortal rays of light divine,
Oblivion to illume bright as this world

By glory-gleaming lamp of day lit up,
Whiles vast of endless gloom night-hidden yet
From mortal sight, I rove by *Vision* led;
That dread unknown of wonder to unveil,
And mysteries beyond the deep grave's brink
By sacred Song divinely to reveal—
Sinners to wake from the dark-death of Sin
(To which compar'd all darkness else is light)
To Virtue's heavenly day, that they may live
To Wisdom,—hand in hand with Duty walk
Religion's paths of piety and peace
To endless life-of-bliss with God in Heaven.

The Closing Scene, in wondrous *Visions* wild
Give me to sing assisted by Thy power
T' sonorous note of tempest-melody,
Or deep-ton'd organ of Eternity
That smites the listless ear of hideous Ghosts
In Den of Night, and stuns the Wo-gnaw'd soul
Of Melancholy, wreck'd, in chamber damn'd.

Full on my downy couch at eventide
I lay me wearisome. Night's dull-ey'd god

In balmy arms embrac'd a hemisphere.
To death-like stillness hush'd the busy hum
Of men. The Miser, talking o'er gold bags
Till soul's delight to painful labor turn'd,
Clos'd weary-watching eye and prostrate lay
On yellow-hoards, and dream'd that Mammon was
The universe. Dread Midnight came—all gloom!
Look'd o'er his staff with frown Cimmerian;
Grim Darkness felt, down-pouring from his face
Night's noon—allusive of Eternity!
His iron tongue told twelve. Great Nature closed
Her eye,—in arms of dreamless Stillness sank
With noiseless finger press'd to breathless lip
Of Quietness. But still I slumber'd not—
Sleep was denied me! Untold burdens crush'd
My spirit-tower, and hurl'd from bosom's god
Heaven-breathing Peace, and gave my heart to wo.
Rolling and toss'd by Restlessness I lay
Impatient quite for death-desir'd and sweet
Oblivion, from tortur'd Thoughtfulness
All earthly ills to chase, and plunge to deep
Forgetfulness life-woes—sin-wounds of soul!
Care-breeding Time had given; when orient

To spirit-sight—all-seeing VISION came!
Her wing celestial plum'd, and to me gave
The Valley of the Shade of Death! Roll'd up
The curtain dark of Doom. Mind's startl'd eye
Affrighted sore, drank in—Eternal Scenes!

Half way from Earth—that busy stage of Man!
From Heaven, too, and fiend-howling Hell half
way,
Pois'd 'like by all and equally remote—
A World of Wonder leap'd before my sight!
Where Night Eternal plumes her dragon-wing
O'er Horror's wastes and Melancholy's seas,
That fill'd all space 'twixt Chaos increate
And Being's bounds: it was—OBLIVION'S VALE.
One rageless terror all alive with deaths!
Where silver moon, nor planet's ray, nor morn
Nor day, with Heaven's life-giving smile may
come
The brow of black Despair with light to crown
And unto Desolation desolate
New being give whiles endless ages roll.
Blackness of Darkness mighty on her wings

Broods on eternal and eternal frowns
Gloom frightful, killing Mist and deadly Shade
O'er regions dark and Shadow foul of Death
Where Ruin wide with Midnight Darkness stalks
Thro' Silence' halls and fell Destruction's home.

No life is here! No happiness, no joy;
No love-enamor'd youth and sweet-lip'd maid
That live and feast upon the nectar-kiss
Stray thro' the mournful desolation vast:—
Love's eye hath lost its fire, his cheek its smile,
And song of Mirth is hush'd by mourning Wo,
The nimble-footed Dance by trembling Age—
A stranger Sport, and Pleasure never known!
Nor voice hath Joy, nor smile Festivity,
Sunshine of Affluence cloud-obscurity—
E'en Hope lies bleeding vanquished by Despair!
Here Slumber sleeps with dreamless Quietude,
While Spirit wings its sentence to receive—
To bask in glory or to rave in fire.

No giant Forests robed in living green,
Like mighty armies stand majestic here

The Storm-clouds battling for a century.
No Muse-inspired Wood, to wake the Breeze
To all the melting melody of Song,
And woo the Dew-drop from her heaven-high
home
And wed her to his flowery breast till morn.
Nor towering Oak, with cloud-uplifting head
To bid defiance to the raging Storm,—
To cradle fiery Lightning in his arms,
And hush to quiet, bellowing Thunder's roar,
Whiles giant bosom lulls to sleep profound!
Or Mountain Fir! to wave sublime her arms
Of fadeless green and head immortal, high
'Mid Ether's home! and play at will and mock
The wasteful Whirlwind in his battle-car
Sweeping in might and thundering in his ire,
And lash the scolding fury into calm.
Nor whispering Grove, nor love-inviting Dale,
Or Mead where Violets sip fresh tears of Dawn
And sunbeams lend their beauty to the rose,
Wake Zephyr's lute to melodies of Heaven.
Or Grot, or Glen where Love breathes wedlock-
vows

While bright-eyed Eve high sits her star-gem'd throne
And feeds the thirsty Flowers with balmy dew
'Hind curtains fair of oriental Day.
No crystal Brook—no heaven-reflecting Pool
Where fishes show their silvery sides in sport,—
Nor Nightshade, nor the baneful Hemlock grows,
But unto mountain-flights—towers *Dust* instead
That Death's right arm of strength had robb'd of life
And hurl'd from Earth six thousand years ago.

No Spring to wake her little infants up!
No Summer paints her blushings on the pink
And rose's cheek, or heavens the violet's lip;
Nor yellow Autumn breathes to ripe her fruit,
Or view her leafy-honors fly the breeze,
But Winter reigns sole monarch of the year.

No crowing cock tells day's awakening hour;
No feather'd songster hymns of rapture sings,—
Not e'en the sombre raven croaks his song,
Or hoarsely hoots the ominous bird of night,

But all is silence felt—Oblivion!
Where Stillness stands with finger to his lip
A-hush, aghast—voiceless, nor dares to breathe!
While brooding Melancholy ever reigns
Quiet as death and solemn as the grave.

No cities vast to boast of massive gates
To many walls of hundred steeples high;
Nor man, nor beast, nor any thing that lives
Or moves upon the flowery Earth that eye
Hath ever seen, or ear heard is here;
'Tis wonder all and mystery yet unveil'd
To spirit-sight—Eternity alone!
Ne'er see can Life, man living never know:—
What *living* ye know not, *dying* shall know,
Nor then, but this: What is—E-T-E-R-N-I-T-Y!
E-ter-ni-ty! Enough for Saints to know—
Eternity can know Eternity.

How awful, silent, vast, is this dread world!
Above, below, around—leaping all bounds
'Tis one vast wild of solitude and night,
Immensity of loneliness and death

Bordering the horrors of Infernal-world!
One dismal void of Emptiness and Nought—
Amaze and lifeless-night—Oblivion!

O, Universe of Wonder and Dismay!
Region of Shadow and of doleful Shade!
Gloom-wilderness and cave forlorn of death!
Sin-frown and Devastation's reign supreme!
Chaos-confusion—end of ruin void—
The home of nothing, yet—the home of all!
The shuddering blank of Grim Forgetfulness
Where thought is lost as wand'ring Chaos-wilds,
And dismal Night and endless Quiet lower
Dense-darkness Day-god's fires could ne'er illume!
Where Wind lives not, nor Storm is known to
breathe;
Where Whirlwind sleeps and Tempest is not
found—
E'en the light-coated, silent-tripping Breeze
And Zephyrus stand dumb as Silence' self
And—eating their own breath! All is—Death's
hour!
Forever-more is frightful Vacuum,

Eternal Stillness and the deadly Damps—
Fell Desolation and Nonentity!

This is *Eternity's* lorn home of gloom,
Dread home, and by him call'd—'*Oblivion's Vale.*'
Mausoleum of Nature's every dust,
Where all Earth's ashes sleep—a harmless pile,—
Together mingle friendly and beloved
With Peace and Quietude till Judgment-dawn
To life and immortality shall wake.
Eternity's long, long-lone bed of sleep!
Where all mankind (Sleep's own true votaries)
Eternity shall find filling desire.
That bed, already made, calls loud for Man,
And Death awaits to lull him to repose
Till Gabriel's trump with jarring sound shall rend
Creation huge, and all her massive Worlds
From their deep-rooted spheres shall fall head-
long!
O, drowsy mortals—wake! to duty rise
While yet arise, while yet awake ye may,
And tremble at the voice that calls ye hence,—
Ye wicked—tremble! all ye righteous—smile!

Now, all Oblivion roll'd before my sight,
And Night-frowns dismal and Death-vallies look'd,
All stirless, breathless, soulless solitude—
Oblivion! it lay huge—lengthened out!
Eye-straining heights down to sight-loosing
depths—
Infinity's flight-boundless, countless width!
As wild and lone—sear too and terrible
As great Sahara is whiles Simoon rolls
His hell-car on to gorge whole caravans
Of Arabs at a meal! Around I gazed
But nothing saw save Death's down-crumbling heaps
Mould'ring in ruin. Cell to cell and cave
To cavern gaping deep profounds. Dungeons
And labyrinths of wo—mad'ning to thought!
Many a ruinous, many a craggy maze
Of dismal Ruin frowning peril 'round!
Bays lash'd to waves and inward-groaning lakes.
Ghost-dreariness. Fell Horror's hideousness.
Hell-shade. Pale Fear look'd terror thro' the
gloom!

I saw a *Sea!* Fierce-raging sea and deep,

And wide as deep, and dreadful too as wide!
Oblivion's Vale its fearful billows dash'd—
Dividing vast Eternity from Time,
And Life from Death, the soul from Spirit-land;
Mortality from Immortality—
From Substance, Shadow all, and nam'd—DEATH'S BRINK!
Where waves distracted with distracted waves
Wage war eternal with uproar of Hell,
Whiles Alpine-mountains rise the dwellers dark
Of Limbo-skies! The foamy Brink to depth
Boils like Atlantic's mad, shipwrecking waves
Cloud-pil'd by Storm, and wild Confusion reigns.
In wrestlings hot of rage the gale-born surge
White-leaps, and bounding from loud-roaring rocks
Afar bursts thund'ring and dissolves to foam.
Grim Death, each billow rides exalted high,
And with a life-annihilating look
On like wide waste of Desolation rolls
With Devastation in his grin! While huge
With horrors, wide beneath opes realms of Wo
Mad'ning to thought of less than Angel-mind!

Appalling seems its swell, and Man affrights!
Deep dread to all that live upon the Earth.
But sure, to fallen man it should be sweet
This Brink to cross in bless'd Religion's bark
With all its silken sails for Glory spread!
Tremendous, tho' it even seems to rage
And fur'ous beat and lash and rend the shore
Of Time with jarring sound of horror dread
And wo—it only *seems:* its stunning voice
Of melancholy, as an empty sound
The much-mistaken ear of man alarms—
Like Spirits sent with warnings for our good.
Life's dream is tempest all where death finds calm;
Man thinks it bitter till he tastes it sweet—
Sees Horror only till he's hail'd by Peace!
The good have nought to fear, their loss is gain—
Eternal gain! O, journey most beloved!
The passage pleasure and reward immense.

Wide is the Brink—too wide to see beyond!
Upon its bosom's fiercely heaving swell
I saw a broad-wing'd *Vessel* sweetly glide

By waves untouch'd, unharm'd. Storm held his
breath
At her approach, the mighty billows slept
As she drew near, and mirror'd water's face
Smil'd gentle Calm, love-greeting her in peace.
A gallant Vessel tall, strong, mighty she:
Her timbers, cedars vast from sunny shore
That knoweth no decay, fram'd, finish'd are
With such celestial order all complete
That Beauty spake to Harmony—'*Divine.*'
Her yards the virgin-gold; her air-wed sails
Are as space-losing wings of Spirits bless'd
Bath'd in Redeeming Love and glowing out
And sparkling with the smile of God! E'er
fann'd
By spicy gales of Grace they swell full, round
As moon—nor wind, nor wave adverse, oppose.
Prow adamant, by a celestial hand
Divinely form'd! where pictur'd Loveliness
In beauty pure appears as orient
As Morning's light; and bright Seraphic bands
Grace-form'd, love-cheek'd, blaze thick as stars of
night—

Sunny with halo-floods divine, that days
With Immortality the Heaven of Heavens!
They seem alive—inspired with action, sense
And speech just less than gods, and far above
All grasp of mortal mind. They, glory smile,
And with immortal palms—'*Kind welcomes*' wave
To white-rob'd Purities when forth they leap
From prison-dens of frail Mortality.
Perfection, from her masthead loud proclaims:
'SHIP ZION, built by heavenly Architect.'

For Light-house bound and haven of Repose!
Fleet sailor for Eternal Glory's port—
Sure sailor for bright Eden of our God!
Upon her deck and in her cabin large
Whose floors were gold with diamonds thickly set,
I saw a heavenly band all rob'd in white
Bright as a sun, yet mild as moon full-orb'd
With Heaven's divinity of loveliness.
Each face, with fires celestial lit and love
Eternal, blossom'd out a Paradise
That Eden-bow'rs and Youth Immortal look'd
Majestic, soft, seraphic and God-crown'd!

With soul-rejoicing sound they shouted loud,
Till hymn-re-echoing halls of Old Ship Zion too
Found spirit-voice harmonious as they,
And vocal-joy with speaking-shouts replied;
While Angel-songs and notes of bright Redeem'd,
Roll'd praise melod'ous thro' the Heaven of Heavens
T' Eternal Spirit and the Lamb; amen.

The *wicked*, were not there! They, from the shore
Of Time, Death plung'd headlong in his own Brink—
His boisterous Brink and stormy Sea of Wo
For fiery home in tempest-world of Wrath
Where Hell-of-sulphur rolls without a shore—
Distraction-lash'd and howling hideously!
Where Dying-death lives reigning a proud seat,
And Torment fierce and Vengeance never sleep
While Woe's enormous howl counts years with Hell:
Where mountain-waves as thousand oceans huge
War waves as fell, and hot in fury pour
Perdition manifold—vindictive fire.

Wan Spirit-troops by Wrath Divine pursued,
The wavy Brink hot-speeding o'er, I saw,
In all the sad varieties of wo—
Anguish unutterable deep pondering on
And bitterness of Hell. Beginning now
The harvest dire to reap sins manifold
Have sown: first Hell-smite from Despair's fell frown!
First taste from the gall-brimming cup of Wo!
First death-pang from Undying Worm's dread tooth
Soul-rending sore to endless evermore!
Eternal Wrath's first arrow—drinking spirit!
Destruction's dawn whose woes are Legion all—
All blasting, withering, wasting, countless deaths.
Groanings commenc'd to groan to groan for aye.
Their voice of wail, their howlings of despair,
Infernal growls, annihilating shrieks
One bedlam-roaring wild, horrific made
Storm-loud, and fell as thunder—crushingly!
Whiles their damn'd looks of everlasting grief
Spake spirit-death and soul asunder riv'n
By fell Damnation's fire-claw ruinous

And lightning-wrath of dread Omnipotence.
High o'er the mountain-rolling waves they leap'd
Dash'd, mourn'd and wept and gnash'd their teeth
In misery consummate and ruin damn'd!
Some, plung'd headlong beneath the angry surge
Struggling with death-of-fire flame-gnawing sore
As Death-worm's sting tremendous, convuls'd.
But vain each effort—all their labor vain,
As soon might wash all Ethiopia white
As one lost soul from deep corruption's stain.
And some, lone-wander'd 'mong loud-roaring waves
In deepest gloom—to dumb despair sunk mute
And look'd enormous wo whiles toiling hard
And long and vain to estimate the vast
Immensity of trouble, pain, despair
And agony that in one moment liv'd.
'Twas nonsense all and most absurd and vain;
No tongue can tell, no language can express,
No spirit-mind conceive and no harp sing,—
Imagination's canvass picture forth,
Or Fancy's flight e'er bound the boundless void,
Nor star-computing Wisdom e'er sum up

The vast, the deep afflictions of an hour.
Soul-wreck'd, on boily-billows, darkling burn'd
As sparks in sulphur den of Erebus,
And shrieking out to each their deep, dire tales
Of wretchedness, whiles sin-uproarous Brink
With demon-rush and voice infernal, gave
No heed, but belch'd new torments on its damn'd—
Forlorn in grief and dismal in despair.

Between Death's boist'rous Brink and Shore of
Time
Wide lay—THE VALLEY OF THE SHADE OF DEATH.
Death's shade-land bord'ring the Eternal-world!
Gloom-veil and shroud of Sin that darkling clouds
The coast of Time, and hides from eye of Life
The Wonder-myst'ries of Eternity!
Mad Horror's fen and gulf of Night, where troops
Of Ghosts aghast, pale, gaping flit fire-eyed,
And shrieking vanish in a groan so dire
That caverns of Eternal Night resound!
The shadow of Eternal Night's dread wing
Whose sable rustle is Creation's sigh
And Nature's piteous moan thro' all her works!

Sin-ruin void, Crime-oped at fall of man—
By Disobedience delv'd and Satan's power.
Outcast of Being waste and bare and lone
As skeleton of Death! Desolation's
Sad seat all desolate, where the grim King
Of Terrors like a tempest sits his throne
Of skulls, wide looking desolation round
With Devastation's power—frowning for aye
Annihilation to the heart of Life!

Vale of Affright and Dread—black Shade of
Ghosts!
Where Darkness ever plumes her dragon wings
And Horror's shriek gives terror to Despair.
Two *Roads* I saw. At Gate of Death that wild
Of wo began—'DESTRUCTION'S BROAD ROAD'
call'd—
Death, Hell uniting! Satan's own dismiss'd
From their Sin-vault speed howling. Death Gate
opes.
This Broad Road's hideousness full on their sight
Falls stunningly. Fear-smote roar out the damn'd.
Confusion is and wild uproar—clamor!

They fly—they fall o'erwhelm'd and down plunge
lost
In deadly fangs and jaws of Agony.
They 'scape—they shriek, they howl! and on
speed, leap
O'er fen, or crag, o'er bog—Chaotic-wilds!
Thro' Demon-haunted ravines curs'd from Eld
And 'live with Wretchedness, Wo, Death they
rush
Where Dragons roar and Devils sweep as storm;
While howly Fiends fire-eyed upon them leap
With tempest in their look and wo—mad'ning!
They speed along—confounded speed sin-scourg'd,
While black, grim Night eternal frowns full-faced
With Impy-spectres dangling on each hair!
And Thunder dread from sulphur den beneath
Wakes roar of vengeance and eternal Curse:—
They quake—affrighted fly—shrunk to a groan!
From Death Vale's horrors rise all thunder-
scathed,
Climb rocks—huge as a world! Fell rocks that
shake
As things infirm, and tumble to and fro—

Bend, bow, toss, reel as forests lash'd by storm,
And heart-convuls'd as burning mountains are
When Fire-fiend rends their vitals like a Hell,
Or the Atlantic-isles in Earthquake's grasp.
From peak to peak, from cliff to cliff they leap
Still tow'ring—toiling on and upward still
Unto crag-clad, cave-yawning Mount of Mist
Whose arrow-like flight height-loosing point waves
The canopy of Night rending! Here stand
Wail-voic'd, fell, ravy, fierce—battling Despair
Till flames volcanic meet them and ingulf,
And with Niagara-voice and Malstrom-roar
To Depth's profound hurl spirit-crushingly,
Where fell Damnation waits the soul's death-plunge
To Wrath Infernal—glaring out Hell-fire!
Here, Shadows fierce of grim Departed Joys
Meet every view with loosing gape and grin
Of devils damn'd, while huge in every groan
And mad'ning lives and raves Eternal Death.
Rage-lash'd and horror-struck, look—death of wo!
Thro' Den of Spectres rush—thro' Gloom of Doubt—

Pass Terror's Wilds and Fear's and pale Affright's
And Desperation's Cave ope to devour.
Then Shade of Dread and the Undying Worm;
Life's Wreck where green Remorse sits stupefied,
And Horror's Fen reflecting Hell, where fierce
Screams palsy-smitten Shadow of Despair.
Cloud-rangling, here, arise to Chaos Mist—
Death Cliffs! high o'er Destruction's Cavern-home
And Devastation's morbid Den lowering,
Where fell Despair awaits Sin's woful plunge,
Then, lastly, thee—*Lake of Eternal Fire.*

The *Righteous*, are not so. Their grave of peace
By Spirits watch'd and hovering Virtues all
Attended, is the love that marries Earth
To Heaven, and saves the Sin-curs'd world from Death
Eternal, in dark Den of Wo. All round
The Christian's Angel-guarded tomb, wide opes—
THE NARROW PATH TO LIFE! where Virtue's smile
Halos Death Shades with light of Deity,

As rosy dawn with twilight blending soft
Or moon in dim eclipse. Life's Narrow Path—
Wide as the world! where cliff with cliff and crag
With crag join like entangling clouds, till mix'd
They roll united all. Great mystery
Of rock—vast myriads yet one! Heavenly
And all of adamant, where ever dwells
Elysium, with song of the Redeem'd,—
Fresh-falling manna from the Tree of Life,
And Life Eternal ripening into bloom.
The God-like Christians blest as men can be
Have little else to do than shouting go
From New-birth on to endless evermore;
Grim Death but opes his iron gate to wake
Them into life of Heaven, and give their cheek
The Eden-rose of Immortality.

I saw a *Cave*—forlorn of wretchedness!
Death Shades have not another like to it,
So gloomy, dark, foul, dreary, desolate—
So huge and wild—Death Valley's horror, groan!
Pil'd mountain-high with dust of Ancient-years—

Ruin's flight and Devastation's reign supreme!
Girt all sides round by wall tremendous, vast
Of human bones—of princes and of kings!
Dried and cemented by the breath of Age—
The mighty labor of six thousand years!
And this is Death's—*Death's own all direful Home*,
Where fell Disease hath birth, and hell-tooth'd Pain
Affliction woke, and tempest-footed Plague
War, Pestilence and Famine learn to live.

Hard by Death's Home is smooth and silvery *Lake*,
Asleep from fall of man till present time
Without a mote or wrinkle on its face,
Unknown to wing of storm, or wind's rough breath,
And looks the surface of a waveless sea:—
DEATH'S MIRROR true, that shows his hollow eye
Eternal Scenes:—*Hell's* mighty agony
Without an end; her deep distress—her vast
Of troubles deep, affliction sore and fell;

Soul-gnawing jaws of fire! her utter wrath
Interminable and deep'ning evermore—
Despair despairing—Darkness dark'ning still!
Her groans, her tears that burn as living fire
And fill with drops of gall sad Sorrow's cup;
Her writhings of Remorse, dire shrieks of Fiends;
Her Demons damn'd and hot Infernals fierce;
Her raging billows and her sulphur flame;
Her desperate grief and everlasting death—
Eternal wo and infinite despair!

It shows him *Heaven*—with all her blessedness!
Where Love and Mercy bask in fount of Life
And sing and shout with full of joy aloud
Eternal praise to God e'er sweet and new
In floods of glory 'round th' eternal throne.
Where Seraph-choirs with Angel-bands converse,
While bright Redeemed in snowy vesture clad
And diamond-crown'd wave palms of victory,
And grasp their deep-toned lyres with love-smiles
strung
From bless'd Redeemer's lip, and on o'er streets
Pearl-gem'd of Zion fair—hymning the Lamb

In all the melting melodies of Heaven.
Shows all the blessedness of that bless'd world!
Her whispering brooks and mildly talking streams;
Her limpid pools and silver-bosom'd lakes;
Her rosy seats of love and bowers of bliss;
Her grassy meads and violet-smiling lawns;
Her downy plains and lotos-laughing vales;
Her sweetly singing groves and landscapes fair;
Her Zephyr-breathing grots, peace-lisping dales
And silk-leaved glens and lily-gardens pure,
With flowery walks by Angel-foot perfum'd,
Where bright, celestial hosts do oft retire
And reap a harvest rich of perfect joy.

It shows him *Earth!* her empires and her k
Her government and laws; her changes all-
Vicissitudes; her life and death, glory
Decay and happiness and misery.
Death's telescope revealing Mystery!
His eye of augury and of knowledge deep
That makes him true philosopher indeed—
Historian and prophet, magi, sage!
His Shadow-glass reflecting every chance

From Nature's birth e'en on until the now—
With mysteries else that sleep in embryo.
And here, that fleeting shade of substance, Earth,
Sheds Fashion's garb and tinsel-mask of base
Deceit, and palsy-struck, with Vanity
And Vice on totters—Fool'ry, Frailty
Outshaming all vile rags of Wretchedness,—
Haunted by Winding-sheets and famin'd Graves
Wide ope around and gaping hideously,
While fierce Disease with death-bells all a-ring
Howl at her heels loud groaning to devour.
This world, the shadow of a shadow seems—
Illusion of false dream, alluring to
Elude the grasp of Life forever-more;
Yet Folly-chas'd from thoughtless Infancy
To dotard Age! if Chance the phantom stays
She 's Hell's enchanting Mammon sent to damn
The soul and body both eternally.
Earth 's like an egg-shell, seeming to be bulk
While all is empty, hollowness within—
Air-bubble full of utter emptiness!
An Ignis-fatuus show of nothingness!
Limbo of phantom-fleeting vacuum!

Gewgaw complete of perfect vanity
Where nought is certain but uncertainty!
A fairy-tale of base absurdities,
Or romance huge, with contradictions full!
A dark enigma never understood!
A worm-wood bower where honey-dews invite—
The honey-cup of Sin with death in it!
The putrid ulcer of Corruption deep
Where Mankind feast themselves to feed grave-worms,
And on Life's fickle hour air-castles build
Whiles they dream it away to wake in death!
A dunce-block vile where all play fool in turn!
Hot-bed that ripes for endless life or death!
Affliction's depth of beggary and want,—
Her gold, by Miser's careful hand pil'd high
Seems fell Corruption's deadly sting, and each
Adorer stings—killing eternally!
Her titles, crowns, appear of nothing worth—
All tatter'd rags on back of Poverty!
Her highest honors splendid vanities,
Or golden fetters fastening on the soul.
Bed of Affliction and the tent of Death

Where friends meet seldom—ever to part soon!
Where Torment fierce torments with Agony,
While slender-arm'd and ghost-gaunt Frailty
High o'er the world her wide dominion spreads
Showing Earth's treasures false as Love's romance!
The brightest hours oft weaving deadliest snares!
Hope, yielding thorns and blighting all her flowers!
Shows Bliss, not found in all the Vale of Tears—
Ocean of bubbles and a world of wo!

I look'd again. Earth was an ocean vast
Of wretchedness. Wo-lash'd roll'd high her waves,
And deaths were in each billow's heave! Direful
The swell, the roar, the rage, the foam; then—burst!
And rose, swell'd, groan'd and rav'd and roar'd and burst
Again—Tornado-lash'd perpetually!
I heard it call'd—'*Life's Stormy Sea of Grief.*'
Tempestuous scene of sighs and groans and tears!

Death's Storm Gulf ever widening with all wo!
Time's Flood on dashing to Eternity!
Where all Mankind embark'd are dashing on
To Spirit-land. Some, ride in ships secure
Well built and mann'd, regarding not the storm—
Guiding each sail and laboring manfully.
But most are reckless, indigent—slothful!
And these, have a sin-canker of the soul
Benumbing all ennobling qualities
Of mind, and chasing Heaven and God from thought—
Lulling to sleep all that is life on earth,
Till Death awakes them with—deep-death of fire.
These, lost on skiffs, canoes, frail barks and crafts
Float ever down life's Stormy Sea of Grief
Without a Pilot—compass to direct,
Barometer to tell the storm, or north's
Fix'd star to guide aright, nor danger see
Tho' in its midst and ready to engulf!
At mercy of a raging Sea all merciless!
At random drifting to a world unknown—
No port design'd, or light-house for a guide!
A frightful Archipelago it seem'd,

All interspers'd with rocks and islands thick
As hundred eyes on Argus' fabled head;
Malstroms are there and fierce-engulfing waves!
But Sin's blind fleets dash on with idiot-grin
Blaspheming in their pride! or else a-play
With swarms of gnats that hum around the
    prow,
Till whirlpool in its wrath meets and devours
With groan of Death and howl of fell Despair,
While they teeth-gnashing plunge to Endless
    Night
With dismal roar of everlasting wo.

Again I look'd. Earth's wide spread bosom was—
One direful *Grave!* whose jaws abysmal oped
To gorge Mortality,—yea all that live,
The *he* and *she* and *it* of the vast world,—
One hill of death and one wide sepulchre!
Death, busy was, nor weary ever grew,
No labor, or fatigue could stay his hand,
Or seas of blood his raging thirst allay.
He rode on every blast, cours'd every path
And stood in place, or side by side with Life,

Whiles every breath hurl'd thousands to the
tomb—
Triumphing o'er the world victorious.
At every door a greedy Grave he dug,
That all who live should fall to him a prey:—
And so they do! all, great and small, feeble
Decrep'd, and those of giant strength, alike,
Stand reeling o'er the deep Grave's brink, and
soon
To take eternal plunge for bliss, or wo.

Mankind, seem'd dangling on a beam of Light,
A ray of mercy from the Heavenly world—
A wandering gleam from the Eternal Day!
Dim miniature of Everlasting Life,
Celestial fibre fine—Free-agency!
By Vision call'd—'THE BRITTLE THREAD OF LIFE.'
Upon it, all Time's precious jewels hung:
A world of glory bright, a world of wo—
Eternity of wonders ever new!
Man, with his all on earth and hope of Heaven—
Each thing that 's sweet, rich, fair and great and
good,—

Desire the most desired, pleasures untold,
Joy inexpressible with glory crown'd,
The spirit's fullness and the soul's own feast—
Supreme of bliss 'bove Angel-harp to tell,
Suspended are on this—this ray of Love
This Heaven-smile Mercy-sent all merciful
To Man—uniting him with Deity!

There-on, Death breath'd,—'twas broken utterly!
Life's race was run,—its troubles slept in peace.
Man's stewardship and his probation closed;
Enough of Earth—all but a *little grave!*
To king and peasant, this great truth 's the same:
Eternity is all and Earth is nought.
A truth divine with heavenly knowledge full—
Beyond all earthly wisdom to conceive,
Where Nature's every idiot may gain
Soul-saving wealth—the wisdom of the skies
That sun-gems brow of Immortality.

While Death, breathes on this wonder all divine,
Its piteous moans make weep the heart of Life!
The death-vibrating cord talks out to soul

In sadness deep and deep solemnity;
Most solemn, mournful ever heard by Man—
Most melancholy ever known on earth,
Or ever struck the tympanum of Time.
With tongue more eloquent than sacred desk,
Oft from deep sleep the sinner it awakes
That dares the thunders of Omnipotence
In all their fiery lightnings terror-crown'd—
Resolv'd to sleep at hazard of his soul!

Heaven holds o'er Brittle Thread of Life, kind
watch
Continually—her smile divine and care.
And Love and Mercy, too, from Zion Hill
A Cherub sent so fair, pure, bright and bless'd
It beggars harp to tell—its constant guard.
No earthly phrase her glory can express,
Or less than Seraph-lyre her beauty sing:
And she—*Man's Guardian Angel ever is.*
And Man, or high, or low, or rich, or poor—
Each one distinct, his own loved Angel hath
From Angel foul of Death protecting all,
That else would life destroy within an hour.

The Brittle Thread of Life, she busy climbs
From morning's smile to morning's smile complete—
Supreme in love, with mercy glowing bright
And smiling o'er all divinely fair;
Whiles *Death*, destruction-arm'd with sore Distress
Pale Grief, blank Horror and outrageous Want,
Affliction fell and canker'd Misery,
Despair, Wo looking Chaos thro' the soul,
And Famine fierce and Pestilence and War
And Poverty and Pain and Wretchedness,
Stalks daily round a-rave to desolate!
And so he would! did not Life's Angel save
And bid Man live his three score years and ten.

So, Earth appears, view'd in this watery-glass—
Death's Mirror true—Oblivion's silvery flood!
That drinketh in all things as Angel-eye,
Nor leaves disguise, nor hypocritic mask
To hide black hearts in robes of Innocence.
In native garb of ugliness reveal'd—
Light-headed, pompous-strutting Foppery!
The swell, the boast of tinsel'd Vanity!

The gaudy show of giddy-grinning Foolery!
Not outside, but the heart of the great world—
The very nakedness and soul of things.
No pomp, no pow'r—minutia most minute!
Unworthy Life's one gaze, or passing thought
Of mortal man hot-hastening to the tomb.

GRIM DEATH! deep read in Augury's black art
Full o'er his Mirror hung brooding as Night,
Thought-sunk to soul of solitude profound
Motionless, mute. His gaze was agony!
Dread Awe, pale Fear and unfledg'd Mystery,
O'er all the Mirror's red'ning face high-leap'd
Proclaiming Wo on coming in their rear:
To Death, of great import—one with his soul.
His bosom's thunder groan'd, and lightning-eye
Down bent its blasting gaze on Wonders all
That came and went eternal in their rounds:
And all seem'd ripe for Glory or for Hell—
Demanding Death to give them to the shades.
Age following Age from Nature's birth e'en on
To Being's end, in gaudy splendors all
Arose to throne of Honor and Renown

To sleep out life with Luxury and Ease—
And bubble-like to deep Oblivion.

Death's Mirror like portentous comet burn'd
Presaging wo to old Iniquity:
To lowest deep it yawn'd—convulsion-shook!
Wave lashing wave in fury rode its face
Till now unlash'd, unmov'd since birth of Time.
Its wailings rent the hollow vaults of Night
And woke the Echoes of Eternity!
High up rose Death hell-smote,—wilderness-look!
Grim darkness all his thoughts wasteful and dire—
Thought-drowning speech a-struggle in his soul!
The tempest of his breast was sea in storm;
His roar Earthquake—flame-eyes volcanic-fires,
When—lo! Death's Mirror woke, leap'd up and
lived!
Found spirit-voice inspir'd and prophesied:

"A TIME, TIMES AND A HALF" are now complete!
Creation-old is giving birth to New:
An Eden, Nature wakes, smiling a bride,
And Man to life and image of his God

And sweet converse and face to face with Him!
Seraphs and Angels busy are on clouds,—
Skies part—clouds roll—the Lord Jehovah comes!
Immortal glory floodeth Earth as Heaven.
Fell Sin hath fled to Hell from whence he came;
Destruction, Pain and Sorrow, Sighs and Groans
And Tears, gone down to grave forgotten quite;
And Wretchedness and Beggary and Want
Are Wretchedness, Begg'ry and Want no more,
But flame as priests in Kingdom of their God.
Behold! Hell opes her fire-jaws ruinous,
Widening for that grim, mortal-satan—Death!
Blue-blazes-robed comes Worm that never dies,
Each fang agrin, writhing in agony—
Thee, Earth-devouring fiend! to grapple damn'd—
Eternal Death complete and Hell Horrors.'

Death, leap'd aloft with terror and alarm—
Begot of Fear and nurtured by Affright!
Distorted features and his blasted mien
Spake Universalian Doubt with hell
Of scruples rack'd,—Annihilation's blight
Upon rose-cheek of Immortality!

While his cloud-face frown'd night of dark despair:
In horrid grin and deadly stare sat Wo,
And Chaos dire of deep confusion look'd,
Or Infidel agaze at Judgment-morn
When Heaven-gates shut and leave him with the damn'd.
His rattling bones with fierce convulsion shook—
A wild, wide waste of desolation!
Then shrank into a thought and lived a groan—
Grief-worm as spirit damn'd in Vision's Vale
'Live with hell-tortures and soul-agony.

The die was cast and he awoke a storm,
Ashamed, chagrin'd to quake at less than God,
And tempest-bosom's rumbling thunders told
Devouring Etna's rage loud groan'd within
Impatient to belch forth consuming fire.
His red eye's whirl out glar'd terrific flame—
A storm-lash'd ocean foamy in his ire!
'What! trembling yet!' he roar'd, 'Shall Death know fear
Till now unknown? Away false trembling—thou!

Thou hellish fear avaunt! heroic souls
Shall never know ye more. Despair shall nerve
My might, and flaming vengeance speed this arm
To such damn'd deeds of everlasting crime
That Sin's own Hell shall blush to look upon.'
He chok'd to silence quite—Tophet of wrath!
Then o'er Death Valley wide all dreadful stalk'd;
His smiting jaws were thunder's desperate crash;
His eye look'd lightning and his breast told storm—
His passion-howl was noise of multitudes!
With indignation fired as Hecla's top,
And Death Vale's Horrors a new horror own'd.

'Death dares to live!' he shriek'd, 'Death will not die—
Infernal Worm not meet—yawn Hell, ingulf
Me rather. I give Man to die, and—Life!
On lives Death lives—will live immortal aye.
I've myriads of myriads devour'd,
And myriads of myriads to come
Shall place Death rival with Eternity.'
He ceas'd, and roll'd an evil eye at shore

Of Time devouringly. Heavens smile was there!
Circumference of Being rose before
His sight a mighty wall—heav'n-high! from deep
Oblivion, and Vale and Shade of Death
Protecting Man for thousand years to come.
Its many towers high-lifted up stood stars,
Where Angels fair and Seraphs bright of God
With eye of love their watchful stations keep
Continually. Death shook, and sighing said:
'Must I to flames and sulphur fire descend?
In every thought a thousand furies rave—
Their shriek is ruin and their howl despair.
How am I driven to extremities!
Awake! the last dread effort shall be done
And Desperation's self be made ashamed.'
He still'd and stood. He shrank into himself
Immers'd, a gloom profound deep pondering—
Apolyon-like! and desperate, deadly all
As sable fiend—Hell was personified!
High o'er Eternal Gulf hung he long lost,
To dismal deep of fell Distraction hurl'd;
His frantic mind uproarous as a sea
Roved all the Den of Wo rent as a world

By Earthquake's rage convuls'd. Thoughts mad-
'ning swarm'd:
A thousand baneful projects struggling rose
Thro' Bedlam-brain all damn'd as Erebus,
And gave a blot to register of Crime.

Thus, self-communing, a long hour he stood
Dreadful as Satan at first view of Hell.
This broken speech then fill'd the ear of Night:
'Illume O, Hope! the deep of my despair—
One beam amid eternity of fears!
Or he, or Death shall die. Can he be slain?
Can Death? I—he—annihilation know?
Exist eternal in yon Gulf of fire!
Stay! both shall reign:—hah! both? Expel him?
So—
My only hope. O, Death! be zealous in
Pursuit as Holy Ardor storming Heaven,
Or Faith unshaken cleaving to her God
While legions of Adversity oppose:—
Hell-fires to fury of grim Vengeance add!
Whatever can be done shall Death not do?
Despair! here end thy moan; assist me—Hell—

Ye impy throng of Pandemonium!
King, father, Satan! Death demandeth help!
I charge thee by the Pit to aid thy son:—
Death, Hell united, all high Heaven shall quake!
To conquer is my life—eternity!
Then stand resolved and vengeance is on wing—
Be firm, and grow immortal by great deeds.
Can Death be slain? the terror and the wreck
Of worlds—devourer, conqueror of all—
The death and grave of all Creation's sons,
Whose home's Oblivion and whose empire Life!
Shall fell Destruction's self no more destroy?
Death lives, tho' great Eternity be wreck'd—
In tortures Hell, and Worm an agony!
I, that my millions daily can devour
And slake my thirst on royal blood of kings,
Must I keep fast for—*a long thousand years,*
Or down to Wo, to Ruin and—Hell-fire!'

Grim Terror lived and king'd the throne of
thought
And chain'd his tongue and lock'd the door of
speech.

He stiffen'd with despair, a-gape—hideous!
An Ocean-grief and vast abyss of night:—
Despair's simoons spread desert thro' his soul!
His slightest look was lightning's fiery glare;
His roar Apolyon's; jaw's crash—crush of worlds!
As gor'd Behemoth desp'rate in his rage
And foam and torture fierce, he o'er the plain
Bounded—stark mad! Around him Midnight lower'd.
Dreadful Tornado sweeping in his might,
Or Whirlwind dire, thund'ring a ruin on—
Sahara was behind him as he fled!
Wasteful as Earthquake jail'd in womb of worlds:
The Vale and Shade of Death to centre shook,—
Infernal Deep reechoed wild uproar!
Death's direful Brink at single bound he leap'd,—
Each stride, Oblivion-hills and Vales forlorn
And solitudes profound behind him fled—
One storm of vengeance blasting as he swept.

BOOK II.

The Closing Scene.

BOOK II.

YET once again celestial Vision came!
Her golden key, Death's brazen door unlock'd
And gave to view unveil'd Eternal Scenes,
And me to wing at will with spirit-speed
Thro' blank Oblivion and Eternal Night.

Death's Brink adjoining, nearest to the world,
Wide, gloomy lay the Fame-devouring Vale
Of GRIM FORGETFULNESS! whose Shadows are
Annihilation—everlasting death.
All things divorced from Life and wed to great
Eternity, here sleep till labors done

On Earth, or good or bad, to right or left
Shall cease to lead mankind, and tongue of
    Fame
To voice their names a speaking echo on
To plaudit of Posterity. And here
Eolian-voic'd Renown with dire Oblivion
E'er struggles for the crown of Glory—vain!
Forgetfulness, with wide chaotic-gape
And look of ruin void as Dante's Hell,—
Fierce too and mighty as his thousand fiends
And spirits damn'd, o'er all that leave on Earth
A blaze of glory or a shade of shame
Triumphs, as Tempest planting forests huge
Amid cloud-land at will, till lost in drear
Oblivion, all mortal things shall one
With nameless shadows be, and onward through
Eternity without a murmur roll.

Beyond, and isthmus-wedded unto Hell,
Confusion lay, and *Shadow of Old Night*,
And *Horror's Vale* embosomed in Despair;
Sad *Sorrow's Pit* and the deep *Den of Wo*
Where Hope dawns not nor Pleasure ever smiles,

But startling Gloom and Cloud and lowering Shade
Jet-mantl'd stalk with chill of death—dismal;
And sore Affright dark dwelling in herself,
At shriek of Ghosts stands stricken and appall'd,
While Horror's blood runs curdling in his veins!
One round of ruin lone, waste, wild, lost, dead
As midnight's dream of Hell that Chaos-like
Comes darkling in its depth of hideousness—
Annihilation opening in its look!
Where Spirit Darkness, out on dragon-wings
Forever broodeth with her weight of death
Brightening with Blackness—sun-eclipsing all,
Whiles Night, chaotic and infernal frowns
Soul-blinding clouds from brow cimmerian
Horrid as Shadows of Nonentity
Lock'd in Death Caverns of Oblivion.
Ten thousand suns here plac'd would rayless be,
And lifeless every Day-awaking smile,—
To Darkness turn'd Creation all a-blaze
And all light quench'd save smile of Deity!

Forlorn in EVIL'S GULF, all mortal things
By Sin and Satan led astray on Earth

And to dumb idols join'd and death, lie wreck'd—
With sense of ill and smitten by Despair.
Ghosts of the Damn'd oft haunt this dire abode
And mourn and howl and curse their body's
dust
That sleep alone for Hell—soon to be burn'd.
This awful Gulf seems dying Wretchedness—
Inert, yet moves—insensible, distress'd!
A secret misery lives in every part—
Unseen affliction breathing thro' the whole!
One wretchedness, one horror and one wo—
The shadow-presence of Eternal Death!
A miniature dim-dawning of Hell-fire
And prototype of suffering without end!

On sped I—spirit! wandering Chaos-wilds
As swift as Angels wing from star to star,
Or thought that leaps Creation at a bound,
While Chaos lower'd on old Cimmerious
Out-darkling Midnight with their horrid beams,
Where things eternal in sleep-dreamless rest
Till dust-awaking-coming of the Lord—
Mortality's own immortality!

Imbosomed in Oblivion's quietude
And quite within the smile of loving Heaven,
The Blood-bought VALLEY OF ELYSIUM lay:—
The Eden bright of dark Oblivion,
And Christian's safe retreat from Death and Wo.
How holy, quiet is their calm repose—
Resting embalm'd with Immortality!
The happy Christians are the lights of Earth,
By righteous deeds with Joys Eternal oned;
Their glory's day shall never have a night.
Home of the Good! bless'd Piety's repose!
Where Virtue's own on bed serene of Peace
Do sweetly sleep with heavenly Quietude!
Their virtue gives perfume unto their dust,
And living light that sacred dust illumes,
Till every atom beams as stars thro' night;
While Valley, all, high on the dome of Heaven
Divinely glows with Glory's halo-flame—
Lustrous as light of Immortality!
No howl of Ghost disturbs their deep repose,
But calmly, they, the Judgment Morn await
Seeming to know their title to the skies.
O, happy dust that sleeps alone for Heaven!

Bless'd rest that waits the coming of its God—
A sacred prelude to eternal Joys!
Heaven's smile e'er showers on them a Father's
love
And joyous sleeps the holy dust of saints.

Between Confusion's Wilds and Eden Vale
Deep sunk to blinding Shadow of Old Night
Where Darkness grim frowns blackness that is
dense,
A cavern hideous and forlorn I saw—
Soul-moving as fire-jaws of Erebus!
Fell Fury's ravy den uproarious, damn'd
Seeming to hate and loathè itself most loath'd—
Ready to burst with wretchedness within!
One ruin void—Oblivion's terror, groan,—
Hell never made nor hath Oblivion seen
A horror helling it! God's frown of wrath
That kills the heart and desolates the soul!
Spirit-despair and Ghost-affright that hurls
Annihilation at Eternity
And thunder-bolts thro' Immortality:
This is the Hadean home of fell—DESPAIR.

Deep sunk to shade of Sadness and Affright
Where Day's one star did never penetrate
Or face of orient Morn hath never smiled—
A Gulf of Darkness roll'd before my sight!
As fierce as Etna hurling forth her fires,
Or mighty Whirlwind's thunder-car, devouring:—
Tumultuous all as giant Malstrom's rage
When thousand whales lie struggling in her womb.
Beyond all oceans wide, all seas in depth—
Despair despairing—black Cimmerius
Dense-darkning still! A wall eternal rose
Encircling vast profound on all sides round
High lifted up, and stood as Horror's wings
Around the bosom of Nonentity,—
E'en towering on to Shadow of gaunt Mist,
And bound Eternal Darkness fast as in
A prison! Whiles on its top of dreadful Night,
Huge mountains upon giant mountain-brows
Lay pil'd like cloud on cloud,—as might of Thought
Sky-towering—towering up and onward still!
Where Fear wing-footed, wed to hiding place

Secure clave close, yet as the aspen quak'd,
And Terror and Affright leap'd breathless on
From crag to crag as silent as the Shades!

Remote in distance dim, a meagre form
With howlings deep—grum, grizzly, now appear'd.
In coming, seemed, all giants Earth e'er knew
Were moulded into one, and that one—he.
Deep awe was 'round him! terror and pale fear—
Soul-losing as grim Death's dark Vale of Skulls;
Wild Wonder's wonder! Dragon-like came dread,—
Enormous, too, as hugest pyramid
Old Egypt all embalming with renown,
That scorns both Ruin and Oblivion,—
Forever named in annals of the world
'Time's Mystery,' all ambitious evermore
To count duration with Eternity!
His stride, Apolyon's shaking Erebus—
Oblivion shook and darkened as he came!
Gloom grew more terrible and Horror's Caves
More dire. Hell's far off roar was heard; Ghosts
    shriek'd
And dismal smote the wailings of the Damn'd.

Deep of Oblivion, down to centre quak'd
And groan'd convuls'd! as hideous as Night-
mare
In madman's brains, and fell and turbulent
As demon-riots fierce in wizzard-wilds.

To Gulf of Darkness drear, all dreadful swept
Roaring as Whirlwind—desperate as Despair!
Whiles his distorted look, Hell-fury glar'd
And fell Damnation's death of agony.
To brow of Night he like a Dragon rose
Fiend-howling and cloud-wing'd, and perch'd—
hideous!
Grim as Destruction pondering ruin stood
With Devastation in death-wilds of thought,
The fires of Hell hot-mingling with his wrath
As Furies fierce—beyond name terrible.

The world's Goliaths vast and Sampsons strong
To him compared contemptuous pigmies are,—
More mighty than Xerxes five millions-arm'd!
Towery his form! A promontory seem'd
That frowns to scorn old Ocean's lashing Tides

And storm-begotten children of the Deep,—
Colossus shading half Oblivion!
His giant shoulders fearful in their strength
Hung massy-huge and broad and round, and might
At will up-heave from fixed foundations firm
The Apennines with all their weight of woods.
His arm of strength, too, wield a thousand oaks,
Or hurl to sky, or snap them all in twain
As boy the cane that dangles at his side.
His hand of bone in its fell grasp of death
Pluck Gibraltar from rock-rooted base
And fling afar to middle of the sea.
His face of storm look'd devastation wide
And age and ruin gnaw'd by Sin and Wo—
Abaddon-deadly hollow of his jaw!
Diseases-millioned, cavern'd in his grin.
His eyes, out flaming anger's wasteful fires,
Like baleful comets from their dreadful orbs
Roll'd fearful wilds of emptiness remote.
Upon his brow dread Vengeance hung and all
The frowns of Night. His Hell-fill'd bosom's core
Like Hecla burn'd with its infernal stores—
Satanic-soul a-struggle to devour!

A raging Ruin and all-smiting Curse,
And vast Oblivion 'neath his fury shook.

Now like some wo-gnaw'd Fiend intent on prey
He forward lean'd him o'er a Dart—hell-tipped!
By Wrath Divine from baneful comet made
That hung nine days and nights o'er Eden-bliss
Proclaiming loud to her—the Fall of Man.
It, red till now, as Lightning's death-glare glow'd
Fiery and fierce to smite continually:—
At near approach of blood, was ever wont
To voice itself high up to Terror's ear
In hollow, wolfish sounds—*now it was still!*
And dumb and dead and ponderous and long—
Like half extinguish'd meteor of the night,
Glow'd wasteful ruin—rageless by his side!
Its barb'd point nesting in his viper-beard
Hid safe, as Fear from coming of her foe.

A Scythe enormous fill'd his right hand's grasp!
A Fury fierce, at fall of man by Sin
And Death and Satan forg'd from sheet of flame
In sulphur den of lowest Erebus.

Nine times the measure of Apolyon's foot
In width the sable vengeance frightful spread,
Ten score in length the hellish ruin gleam'd,—
Lightning its point and thunder was its edge!

In grand divisions, two, the Scythe itself
Divided was: this one call'd—Life, that—Death:
These, subdivided into four, and named
Youth, Infancy and Manhood and Old Age.
And pictur'd on its blade, and prominent
In living characters of fire were seen
All things that den themselves in Satan's soul:
Hell's triumphs and Apolyon's victories;
Sage Lucifer with apple of all ill
Hiding Creation from the smile of God.
Grim Death by Fallen Nature crown'd—half god!
Mark'd Cain with Murder's club that Abel slew,
And Vice and Error and blind Ignorance,
With Superstition and fell Bigotry,—
Dread Vengeance and God-daring Blasphemy;
Fierce Persecution torturing Piety—
All Egypt Plagues that smite Religion sore.

A mighty host was pictured out as life,
Thick peopling a waste-howling wilderness.
Anon, a murmur ran throughout its ranks,
When they did herd themselves together 'round
A head one clamoring: 'Up, and make us gods
To light our paths thro' this dark night of gloom
And untrod wilderness.' Their head, for time
Stood firm,—with noble mien and thundering
brow
Cried—'*Nay.*' But Satan in the hearts of all
The people moved till in fire-words was seen
Assassination near! Submissive bowed
That head:—off broke gold-rings and gave to fire,
When, out straightway all glowing came a—CALF!
Elect ones saw shouting: 'This be our god
Who hath with stretch'd-out hand Omnipotent
His chosen from Egyptian-bondage brought!'
Wedge-like around, the thronging multitudes
Uprush'd admiring; while God's people bow'd
Them down and worship'd all. Arose again,
Peace offerings brought and burnt; then hand in
hand
Around it shouted, played and sung and danced!

While Hell loud bellowed bedlam of applause,
And king Beelzebub in very midst
With mow agape from horn to horn, all like
A Dragon stood, and at their worship—roar'd.

'Bove all upon this fatal Scythe portray'd,
Supremest of the damn'd sat—Lucifer!
By fiery legions throng'd and Death and Wo,
While tide of wrath and biting flames of Hell
Around about with rage infernal dash'd
Startling as crush of a mad cataract.
His look was agony of thought, where sat
Deliberation wild distraction-crown'd;
While his scar'd front in awful pomp upborne
Supreme dominion told and tyrant dread
And unsurpass'd in monarchy of Hell.
Scorn-eyes, full fill'd with flashings of contempt
Flam'd devil-hate; and brows of royal pride,
Majestic and aloft like corners huge
Of worlds, supernal indignation storm'd
Down thundering wide on all the sable damn'd,
And loud to lowest Erebus announc'd:
The king of Darkness—governor of Hell!

'Twas DEATH all dreadful! Chaos of dark night
With Hell's grim Terror-clad and Horrors crown'd.
His gaze was agony—near, 'round, remote,
Await for prey to speak: 'On and devour.'
Wide open flew his jaws to desolate
And belch'd death-plagues to chambers of Despair;
Thoughts madd'ning, all, like fires of Tophet
burn'd:—
He shriek'd aloud! Long, furious and fell
Thro' all the Gulf of Gloom volcanic burst
The hideous clamor and loud raging wail
Disturbing Peace eternized in repose!

As lightning's flash enormous giant rose
All hugeous—ten-score Ghosts a-dangle on
Each hair! He frown'd the Night, and stood
darkling
To Darkness round. No wonder like to him!
So mighty, vast, magnificent and grand
E'en in Oblivion where all wonder is,—
Her mystery, awe, and own astonishment.
He look'd a prodigy—surprising Faith!
All things shrank into nought compared with him—

Immeasurable, incomprehensible
Enigma infinite, Oblivion's
Own lord and king! Array'd in might he tower'd
Omnipotent—Eternity his name.
Vast, boundless, wonderous Eternity!
No Spirit's eye finds centre measuring thee,
And thought no limit to thy dread expanse!

Ghosts at his coming fled aghast, and all
Oblivion bow'd as he arose—cloud-crown'd!
Damnation's Dragons horror-smote at sight,
For refuge plung'd to Pandemonium—
Seeking Annihilation and Inanity!
Confusion with the shock confounded was,
And roll'd through chambers of Nonentity.
Forlorn of Wo felt to her central hell—
Dark-deep-dumb-dead-soul-smitings of Despair!
While all her Furies quak'd, and into arms
Of lifeless Stillness terror-stricken sank,
And silent and death-like with grief-rent souls
On spirit-terror of the scene convers'd.
Fiends vanish'd into Nought, and left—Ruin,
Eyelaying Death with a grim leer malign.

Night in her ebon cell awoke convuls'd,
Bathed locks of long midnight in home of Mist
And Vapor dank, and rustling in her jet
Vanished afar to Shadow, Shade and Gloom
With Spectres damned red-sparkling in her skirts:—
Grim Death hung on the sight—lost—horrified!

Eternity! He had the thunder's voice—
Worlds on fixed orbs, a-jar hung as he spake!
His face of Darkness was Cimmerius;
The chaos of his frown Annihilation,
And Night Eternal in his shadow den'd.
His eyes roll'd Horror-wilds and lightnings shot
And baneful bolts to lowest Erebus.
His arm's fall ruinous—great Being's wreck!
God-like the form he wore—tall as the rocks
That girt him round! Upon his shoulders hung
Smiling, the God-fill'd Heaven replete with bliss,
And frowning, Hell with all its weight of wo.
Yet seemed he incomplete—a part was gone!
Might say—convulsions fierce, or thunder's bolt
Had him in sunder rent in days of Eld,
Or Worm Undying on his vitals fed

For countless scores of years—unfill'd for aye!
In his left side the mighty ruin oped
As many caverns huge 'mong Alpine rocks,
Or ravines wild on maiden Luna's face
By light of Science seen leagues vast in depth.
He, Desolation's wreck look'd desolate—
Ragg'd grandeur and supreme deformity.
Two faces had! opposed as day and night:
In brightness, one, the mid-day sun excell'd,
As other, did in darkness, black midnight:—
Divinity of smiles that spoke of Heaven,
And frowns accurs'd that blasting Horrors told!
With one, he on the Righteous—glory smiled,
And strait they fill'd with Paradise and God;
But other, dark upon the wicked lower'd—
Woe's smite was felt and ruin without end:
Tempestuous clouds storm'd thundering from its
brow—
Each frown distraction look'd and ghost-despair!
Its lightning-flashing eye fierce Terrors roll'd
That zigzag rode Oblivion's vast domain
And to profound of Chaos and Old Night
Red fury glared—ruin hideous and one hell.

Death stood appall'd—perdition in his look!
A Wonder mute and statued Terror dumb
Ingulf'd in wo and ruin manifold.
His speaking look announc'd—'Confusion's depth,
Forlorn of hope and strugglings of Despair!'
And actions, loud as scream of bugle told
Of blight, bane, wreck and desolation all—
Sahara-wide the desert of his soul!
Thoughts mad'ning burn'd and seem'd to desolate;
A Dragon's jargon mutter'd from his throat:—
In all the wilds of deep distraction lost,
Gloomy as Hades dark as Acheron;
Then, with Annihilation's wand seem'd smote
To void of Nothingness—dumb, torpid, dead
As Silence-self sleep-lock'd in bottomless
Oblivion where Melancholy reigns
With utter Stillness and Eternity.
The vast of wonder was—surprise—despair,
And nought save Silence lived! she, lost to self
With Stillness' finger pointing to her lip!
Gloom Vale was quiet as closed sepulchre,
Or Silence' wish breath'd in a prayer to Heaven.

Seal'd, moveless hung gaunt Shadow and wild
Space—
The wailing of Eternal Worm was still!
Dark Bedlam of Despair—inanity,
Damnation's thunder-roar as vacuum!
Nonbeing swallow'd all—forgotten quite,
And action, Motion, Sound suspended were—
All slept! and one death-pause Oblivion was!

Eternal moments pass'd, yet Echo slept—
Voice had no sound! Pale Terror terrified,
Grew stiffning to his place—thought-Agony!
Fear stood vacuity nor dared to breathe,
Affright on tiptoe holding in her breath;
Roar of Eternal Vengeance hush'd an hour,
And universal Nothing seemed to be
Till Death awoke and shook stunn'd and convuls'd,
Then down to hadean-deep of soul he groan'd
Damnation-smote! The Bell Eternal told
One moment all complete while thus he stood
Confusion-fixed and gaping like a hell!
Looking Distraction grinning at Despair
And Desolation in cave desolate.

He turn'd him back from the all horrid Eye!
Whiles in his Legion-heart infernal Wrath
With Furies raved, and shriek'd out thus aloud:
'Hell's furnace in me flames—I am all fire!
Fear blows it up—Confusion and Affright!
Blank Horror, Disappointment and Remorse
Now smite me like a Curse—smite to consume!
Then is annihilation mine—Hell-fire?'
He ceas'd and call'd his Dragons to his aid,—
He call'd on Hell and world Infernal heard!
When, all Oblivion woke, and Horror rose
And Wo with wild Uproar and clamor loud
Of damn'd. Rage, Ruin, Desolation storm'd;
Demoniacs as dismal tempests raged,
And Devils sulphur-robed flam'd many hells—
Burn'd, blaz'd, glar'd, shriek'd till the Eternal frown'd,
And Darkness was—eclipsing Vision's noon!
New scenes oped giving terror to the soul
And blindness even unto Spirit-sight!

Eternity, majestic stood—terrible!
His eye's devouring-stare spake vast surprise,

Whiles his Wrath-face where Vengeance hath his
home
And Horror a proud seat, down poured on Death
Hell-storms! And frowning one eternal night
Spread Chaos out and Darkness dens'd afar!
E'en dim white clouds his face-celestial wore
Thro' which Divinity look'd half eclipsed!
Through-seeing gaze read thought in embryo
And like a tempest he in thunder spake:

'Lo! when there was no Earth save sea, no breath
Save wind, no life save angry water's rush,
Ay, being none but dread Omnipotence—
I was! Infinitude my empire then
And Chaos my domain. Billions of years
Untold, the monarch o'er Oblivion's Vale
I've reign'd, throne, crown and soul, nor rival
found—
Intruding bravo e'en to question my
Sovereignty. Whom see I now? Who dares
Disturb deep quiet of my hallowed home?
Speak—monster! who, and what art thou—thy
name?

What wouldst thy sun-bleach'd jaw's devouring
gape?
Whence comest thou and goest, and wherefore?
speak.'

Death stood all ear in drinking words that burn'd;
Then dwelt apart, and thus to self he spake,
Steeling his mighty heart for battle fell:

'Despair 's in pathway of my brightest hope!
But Death shall courage take e'en from despair:—
Up thou great soul of hell! hast need of all
Thy valor now. Thou heart of many fiends!
Grow one with Desolation's mighty soul:
I charge thee, Death! resolve to do, or die.
To die's to fail, but to succeed is life,—
To live kings Death o'er all Oblivion now:
O, courage take! for wherefore should Death fear?
Fear, I shake off, and trembling shall avaunt,
I bid you fly to Hell from whence you came,
Death needs you not—bane of heroic souls—
The worst of foes e'er met this side Despair.
The conqueror of all will tremble not;

I've been great Being's groan and grave of Life,
Hurl'd Nations down to Ruin and shook stars,
Depopulated Worlds—should I know fear?
O'er Earth and combined millions I've triumph'd,
Her hugest slain, her mighty trod to dust;
Her heroes of renown and Ogres fierce
Before me fell and vanish'd like a dream;
And all with whom I ever did contend
All, all were weak as Frailty to me.
He that can play at will with lion's might,
At leisure sport with hot volcanic fire
And laugh to scorn the thunderbolts of Heaven
Shall not fear less than power Omnipotent!
Omnipotence I grappled with of old,—
With what success? did I not Him o'ercome?
As I do recollect me well—I did!
Victorious. And it was on this wise:
God bade one righteous Noah build a ship,
And on hell-peopled Earth down pour'd a Flood—
Oblivion's winding-sheet and Nature's tomb!
In this wide pall the giant World was wrap'd,
And all things perish'd—man, beast, creeping
thing,

Ay, all save only Death and one lone—Ark,—
An Ark preserved by the Almighty-hand!
To board high Heaven's life-boat I was denied—
Left with Creation's wreck to perish—die!
I scorn'd the Tyrant dread that gave command,
While on a whale's firm back I compass'd Earth
Around—around! and o'er the drowned wreck
And great Omnipotence that ruled the storm,
Thrice shouted I aloud—victory complete.
That was a time! When the high-rolling waves
Down-crushing vengeance of that mountain-mass
And hunger-rumbling bowels of great deep
With all my Woes loud howled in unison!
Whiles Hell and Death triumph'd o'er Earth and
    Heaven—
One carnage made—Mortality devoured!
Yea, I have wared with Him whom none can look
Upon save thro' veiled Vision and yet live!
And I will war—eternal let it be.
Hah! when He sent his Son! His only Son
Of Mary born in ancient Bethlehem,
I hailed Earth's Savior and the Prince of Peace
As devils do damn'd ghosts in world below:

I seized Messias—nailed Him to the cross,
I bow'd His head and bade Him yield the Ghost
And Lord of Glory slept in Joseph's tomb!
Who dares oppose my might unconquer'd? None.
O! when the whirlwind of Death's passion smites
There's nought withstands its wasteful thunderbolt!
Then why despond? Despond not I, nor fear.
Great soul—up! thou my tower of safety be—
And arm! be thou my strength—ye nerves be steel!
Grow firm heart! Bosom turn to adamant—
And Valor! breathe thy calm to Trouble's mind.
Grim Vengeance! one thee now with Scythe of
Death,—
Thou Fury! pour hell-fire in spirit of my Dart—
Arouse thee Death! thy war with giants is.
One blow, Death never aim'd that did not strike,
Nor will, tho' dread Eternity the mark!
A universal conqueror I'll be.
I take mine aim and all things reel around,
I shoot—they fall and all's Oblivion.
Ye high Immortals tremble—tremble ye!
Death as immortal is—your foe for aye.
I am all fire! I'd pluck down firm-fixed Heaven!

Death hath awoke—his strength almighty woke,
Then deeds of desperation are at hand.
The thunderbolt hangs silent—would have wing!
Oblivion! Ho! I'll reign the king of thee
Till God's Millennial Day shall sink to Night
And her wan ghost howls o'er Eternal-hills!
Why thus to self do I soliloquize?
My bellow 's loud above the thunder's roar.

'I face thee—Tyrant! I—Hell's comet fell,
Breathing destruction sure to all that live!
Hah! doth my fury's flame light up these
caves,
And glimmer thus thy cheek ne'er lit before?
I would annihilation was my look,
Thou shouldst be Chaos then as quick as thought,
And I, Oblivion's crown'd instead of thee.
My sun-bleach'd jaws seek—Blood! They will
have blood;
From Earth they come to gorge Oblivion's blood:
My name behold!' His fatal Scythe within
His bony grasp as many lightnings flamed
An hunger'd to devour. He whirl'd it high;

Thro' all the Gulf of Horror and of Gloom,
Infernal flash'd the burning words—GRIM DEATH.

The vast of Darkness shook, dimn'd, paled—lightning'd!
Wide dappl'd o'er with dark and sulphur flame
Confusion-fill'd, hung all Oblivion round
With groanings loud of wo and sullen wrath.
Eternity stood Horror-crown'd complete,
And fierce Damnation struggled in his look!
A weight of night from each dark feature hung,
And Chaos blacken'd where his storm-frown fell.
Throughout his soul's vast desolation throng'd
Wild images of Wo, Confusion dread
Nought, Emptiness, Uncertainty and Doom.
His broken accents long repeated—'*Death!*'
When mem'ry king'd the throne of mind he spake.

'My servant—thou! The constant foe of Life—
The scythe-arm'd Angel of Destruction—Death!
Yon world call'd Earth, now lorded o'er by Time,
Sublimely roll'd with wondrous whirl by long
Lost child of mine around his throne the sun,

Of countless thousands thou dost yearly rob
To gem with sacred dust beyond all price
These vaults inane. My service to thee, Death!
Thou, humble until now, low-bowing cam'st
As servant should submissive, gentle, meek:
Why frown'st thou, Death? Why gaping ruin say?
Why all this mighty storm of burning words?
Why such wing-footed tempest of fierce rage
So loud and boisterous that I knew thee not,
But dream'd of some distracted goblin fierce,
Or demon damn'd from Sulphur-den escap'd
Rent with infernal torture and dire agony?
And thou art angry, mad, enrag'd at what?
I give Grim Death advice,—now listen slave:
Be angry only at thine own misdeeds,
That in thine anger thou mayest never err:
At thine own anger, then, be angry thou
And slay outright; 'twill whet a dart to give
E'en Death his death-wound. Passion, like sea-wave
Swells, foams to burst, and deep to ruin plunge;
But safety, is, where Silence chains her tongue
And holds in bonds the fury of her rage.'

He ended his harangue and frown'd the Night.
Death stood a-gloom, yet preaching to his soul:
All desperate deeds achiev'd in olden time,
All bloody fields his valor ever won,
Thick-crowded on his busy-laboring mind
As autumn's leaves in Borea's chilly blast,
Till light of Reason and Experience proved
Himself immortal and invulnerable.
Then storm'd he fierce, impetuous and proud;
In full glare flash'd his comet-blazing eyes
And deep from Hadean-sockets roll'd—Terrors!
His rage was now a flame that burn'd, his wrath
Fierce desolating fires—thundery in ruin!
He, many devils seem'd—uproarous, damn'd,
And sternly grasp'd his Dart and bellow'd—'Blood!'
When in hot haste Eternity replied:

'Hah! Blood is thy demand! The name's unknown—
Unheard of word in the Eternal World:
She hath no blood for the Devourer's jaws,
Or if she had, where is thy tongue to lap
Cerberian dog of Hell? Wretch'd Man's thy prey,

And Fallen Nature 's a fit mark for thee
Whose being 's but a breath and life an hour.
Thou grim Destroyer of Mortality!
How Satan-like is thy attack on man?
In secret kill'st, and none can hinder thee—
Conceal'd, and massacreing all mankind,
And no one knows aught of the enemy!
To hide in ambush speaks a coward wretch—
Night-hidden like a villain leap to slay!
Full front to front in battle heroes stand,
And the God-favor'd 's crown'd with victory;
But into darkness, Murder skulks away
And base as Hell slays Innocence asleep!
If great, throw off thy cloak of darkness vile—
Reveal thyself, and stand a noble foe.
Dost fear to war with Mortals face to face?
Then dare you brave the fury of my ire?
Thou Ruin-grinning Erebus of Sin—
Avaunt—away! Leave my domain of Rest
Or down to realms of Wo I'll hurl thee damn'd
Mid plenty there to fast eternally
Where Vengeance opes a wider Hell than thee.'

The direful wonder ceas'd, horrific stood:
Huge thunder on his brow show'd storm within;
His eyes glared fury, and loud spake his frown
As tempest-ocean—Ruin look'd afar.
Yet Death stood firm, and widening still his grin!
All fearless his response—impetuous, loud:

'Go bellow thou to Caverns of Despair,
And roar thy stern commands in ear of damn'd,
My jaws I close by swallowing thee and thine.
The fires of Vengeance, Famine burn my heart,
And blood of vast Oblivion shall quench.
Thou frightful bugbear keeping Time in awe!
I'll grapple with thee as in jest, and hurl
Thee forth headlong to Heaven-wed Earth, to blast
Creation with thy presence felt, and give
A blight to God's Millennium! Blood—blood!
I will have blood—Oblivion's blood, and—thine.'
He ceas'd; but his dark brow portending storm
Loud thundered on, and long, tho' tongue was still.
Bold as a god of Eternity replied:

'I'll give thee blood—a Universe of blood!
Take you round Earth! There's blood enough—
the all
Devouring jaws of Hell could ask no more;
To Life's own time-wide scenes of carnage fly,—
Creation's self to heap of ruin hurl
And drain thou dry the rosy veins of Life.
All Nations gorge, and feed on infant's blood
And suck the marrow from the bones of kings:
There too—the Queen! on lap of down soft rock'd,
Her blood of sweatmeats made—delicious meal!
'Twill make the flesh grow thick o'er thy cold
bones,—
Ah! fly thou—fly! the fat'ning feast is thine.'
Death, fierce with fury bellowed out aloud:

'Earth is too small a field for rage so vast
As mine to grapple with—I would have Worlds!
And all the harvest rich of all the spheres
Alone can chase fell Famine from my jaws.
Not ocean, roll'd thro' this hell-heart of mine
Its fiery vengeance would allay, or quench
My fury's rage that sweeps omnipotent

Cloud-shaking thus to dome of Ancient Night!
Ho! I could drink e'en all the blood of all
Oblivion now, and be no jot appeased!
My hunger is a fire! the more 'tis fed
The more voracious gnaws fell Famine's tooth,
And wider flies my Earth-entombing jaws
With louder yells—'Blood! blood!' continually;
So, Ocean drinks Earth's sea-like rivers dry
And roars aloud—'More! more!' perpetually:—
Can endless feasting fill an endless void?
Grim Death is but a famine at full feasts.
Fell Hunger's fangs I feel—infernal thirst!
All things I'll make mine own and then devour.
Begin I will with thee—Oblivion!
And my first meal Time's awe—Eternity!
I feel thee as a morsel in my maw—
And thou art gone and I a-hunger still!
Not Heaven's great Flood from wide oped windows pour'd
World-drowningly upon rebellious Eld
Could fill this maw—immeasurable as Sheol!
To Death's grim jaws all inexorable,
Great Neptune's oceans, seas are but as drops,—

They open without limit—limitless!
They stand as Hadean gates that mock Despair,
And grinning Chaos at the throne of God.
Then sweep to vengeance—Death! and feast thy soul
On Ruin's heart, and fill thyself with wo:—
To conquest—on! Oblivion is a wreck
And Desolation's self more desolate.
Stand thou on guard Ghost-king—Eternity
Grim Death down hurls destruction like a storm,—
Keep watch! my coming is the wo of Worlds.'

He ceas'd. His rumbling throat still rattled—
'Blood!'
Hell-fury bent his brow with thunderbolts.
He sternly grasp'd his dreadful Dart and shook
The wasting vengeance flaming terribly!
He rais'd his pow'r-nerved arm and level'd it;
Back drew afar and frightfully to hurl:

Eternal-arm down fell world-crushingly
And struck the barbed-terror from his grasp!
From Den of Night to Chambers of Despair
In deadly length along the ruin lay

Levell'd with Depth's dark bottomless profound.
Grim Death, Confusion sore-confounded stood,—
He wore Annihilation in his look
Chaos and Devastation in his grin!
Gloom-thoughts storm'd thick, night-black'ning in
his brain;
But Indignation fell and Desperation woke:
Eye's lightnings, smote, and brow hung thunder-
bent—
Rage was at full! And soul-deep burn'd the hell
Of fury that volcanic flam'd in him.
But great Eternity, from deep of his
Divine disgust, knit his storm-face to frowns,
And sat huge Scorn thereon and withering Hate
That call'd Life's foe—'An object of contempt!'
The thunders of his brow struck killingly,
And these bold words from his harsh, hoarse,
rough throat
Like tempests 'round Death's ear roar'd deaf-
'ningly:

'Thou wreck of Ages and of Empires—Death!
Hell-dragon cloth'd by Fallen Nature's rags!

Life-terror and dread enemy of Man—
Destroyer grim! Thy power is measur'd now
As with a span; thy day of cruelties
A tale that 's told; thyself but a sealed book!
Eternal Wrath, is all a-groan e'en now
To light Infernal fires with hells like thee.
Thou mortal-Satan—Death! Why—up and strike!
'Tis nought to me tho' poisonous be thy Dart
And sharp thy Scythe, I can oppose thy might
And stand unhurt defying thee and Hell.
I saw Creation out of Nothing leap,
And I, that honored matron shall behold
Love-nested in the arms of God expire.
These eyes that once beheld young Nature doff
The swadling bands of Chaos and Old Night
Wake Beauty's heaven—put God-like glories on,
Do gaze upon her still and no jot dimn'd!
And Death, that imp accurs'd by Satan got
And born of Sin at fall of man, I'll see
In winding-sheet of World-consuming fire,
And hurl'd to Hell—with Death Eternal oned.
Existence is a cipher unto me,

From stars' first twinkle to their fall as nought;
Time hangs a mote and trembling in my sight,
Creation but a speck and shall have end.
Huge Systems rise and flourish and away,
But self-complete e'er stands Eternity—
Eternity the same eternally!
Before beginning and beyond all end—
The end of every end without an end!
The mighty sovereign of Futurity,
Exhaustless, measureless Infinitude
Without diameter, circumference—
Incomprehensible as God himself!
And who shall talk to me of chance and change?
Let all of vast Existence stand appall'd—
Hell groan, Oblivion quake and Death be dumb.'

He ceas'd to speak. Scorn-frowns thick-tumbling
down
His wrath-bent brow on roll'd wide scattering—
Plagues!
Infernal Pride, Conceit Sin-thron'd august,
From demon heart of Death fell thunderstruck,
And once again his bendless spirit quak'd!

All thought he stood long lost, and look'd a wreck—
Supreme distraction and confusion's blank
Night-lowering o'er the grave of all his hopes.
But nerved by Desperation on, he lit
At Fury's forge the flames of Rage anew:—
Despair-prop'd, inexorable he stood
A solitude of wo and dreadfulness
Like Satan armying all Heaven against
Omnipotence—drinking the dim of hope!
A night of Horrors hung around his brow,
And in his look was all Oblivion seen.
At hand was Vengeance! Ruin woke and lived,
And gave hell-fire to furies of his rage.
Now, lightning eyes met eyes blasting as they:—
Death, howling, swung with rainbow-circle vast
And high to dome of Night, Scythe ruinous—
A-sparkle with Damnation's fiery glare,
Whiles Darkness trembled to her centre Hades
And Desolation echoed from afar!

Eternity, on roll'd cloud-veiled, God-arm'd.
With ghastly grin and horrid stare, Grim Death

Eyed Victory in dim-dawn of Hope, and all
His bones loud rattled out fiend-growlingly,
Whiles round him Shades of Night Eternal hung
Hell-rob'd with every Wo and Hideousness:—
Scenes past seen only in eternity;
Sights, mortal eye ne'er drank with wonder in,—
By flame-eyed Spirits not till now beheld
Divine illumed by Beatific Vision.

Eternity, now smote Oblivion thrice,
And Vision gazed on Emptiness and Nought.

BOOK III.

The Closing Scene.

BOOK III.

VISION, again, gave Spirit to the Shades!
To thee, dire gaping Gulf—thou awful Blank
And shuddering Void—*Oblivion*, Night-crown'd!
Embodied Darkness horrible and lone
Where all is death and space, cloud, shade, mist,
    gloom
And dust and night and ruin and decay
With Desolation's reign without a bound,
While scenes of Wo give terror to the soul
Death-depth chaotic and all bottomless!
The hell of Ruin and profound of Calm,
Where Silence lives and dreamless Nothing *is!*

Where Slumber sleeps till being is entomb'd,
And Dust awakes its sentence to receive
To live in Glory, or to die in fire.

Death Valley peaceful rested with her dust!
Oblivion lock'd the chambers of Repose,
And Quiet sat pavilion'd in her soul.
No shriek of Ghost disturb'd her reign of Peace,
Nor aught awoke her night without a morn.
OBLIVION! Spirit hath not breath'd on thee!
Nonentity that never look'd on God!
Confusion's vast of emptiness confused
With brooding Midnight in her dragon-wings!
All tongueless, breathless, soulless Nothingness
That never gave thought shape, or voice a sound
Wild-shadowing forth death-muteness, tomb-repose!
One long, lone pause supreme—fearfully still,
Soul-smiting, dread as Guilt's lorn dream of Hell.

A *Gulf*, deep-yawning opened to my sight,
All-famin'd like a Grave whose every wish
Is to devour Existence at a meal—
GULF OF ETERNAL RUIN AND DESPAIR!

Infernal Hunger gnaw'd and all agroan
To gore Creation's heart eternally!
Blank Desolation desolate! as huge
As universe and deep as Heaven is high.
Where sickening Mist, Ghost-gloom and Vapor
dank
Shroud Spirits damn'd 'hind curtains of Despair.
The depth profound of void Obscurity
And soul of Night that never dream'd Day *is.*
A condens'd Blackness light could ne'er illume—
Smiting to soul and sun-eclipsing all!
Grim Horror's borders of Infernal World—
Blackness of Darkness Night Eternal curs'd
Dimning to spirit-sight! Darkness and death!
Such, triple-headed Dog at gates of Wo
Would think it Hell-delight, and worthy Sin's
Death-shriek to welcome one damn'd spirit in.

Wide o'er this Gulf of every hideousness,
As Silence pondering, hung—Eternity!
His Tophet-eyes soul-fury flamed around—
On dreadful roll'd the fiery floods remote,
And down afar thro' awful gloom profound

Their lightning-sheeted Terrors redning flash'd—
Chaos was illum'd! Eternal Organ
Peal'd out to Night of—'Resurrection near—
God's Worldquake-coming and the great Assize!'
Annihilating gaze fed greedily,
And secrets all of deep-dark Gulf devoured.
Back turn'd, and shook his sable brows, and spake:

'This gloom looks deadly-fit for Death's abode!
Grim Death! vile fiend sprung from Pollution's mire
To be Life's pest, Time's end—the blank of all.
Thou plague-spot foul on Beauty's cheek of charms!
Mortality's death-smite and Being's grave!
Gall-drop of every sweet upon the earth!
Vile canker-worm within the heart of Bliss!
The burning sigh and groan of Man's loud laugh!
Deep shriek of Misery and loud yell of Grief!
A loathsome stench 'mid Eden of perfumes!
Blot on fair Nature's page! Creation's wreck!
Night of each day! Beginning's final pause!
The grave-mouth'd Erebus of Mortal things,
And coffin-tongu'd devourer of the world!
How many roads to his abysmal jaws

And all horrific! Drinks--is ever dry,—
Blood-drunk, and yet athirst for Oceans still!
World-gorging, yet eternal-hunger gnaw'd!

He stands teeth-gnashing, cavern'd with Despair
And lost in mighty desert of his soul!
Distraction's Spectres fill his midnight mind.
Anguish arave in heart of Wretchedness—
Rending to spirit! Soul of Tophet he
Whose groaning shriek—'Hope hath no being here!'
Grief, Torture and Remorse him hellward bend
A complicated horror consummate.
Screams, yells speak out what tongue of Agony
Can name. Ah! what the core of heart's wo now!
He stands a statued Death a-gape at Wo;
Plague, Famine, Pestilence den in his jaws—
Hell-grin! His voice gives out a prison sound.

'He raves! A thousand deaths are in his frown,—
Night blacks 'round him—Damnation 's in his thoughts!
Above, about him lowering tempests hang:—

Despair! He grapples with Despair in her
Own den loud shrieking—Blood! Fire-eyes roll
deaths,—
Flame-eyed as Vengeance looking Torment's woes
Thro' souls of Furies fierce and Dragons damn'd.
In battle fell and devil-howling join'd!
Their wrath-fires burn. Their wasteful rage devours.
They many Demons seem—thunderous in might!
Dreadful as Heaven's own storm-creating Wrath
Smiting with thunders huge Leviathan.
Horror! Despair to Hell down hurl'd—headlong!
While caves Eternal echo from afar
And world Infernal 's a death-agony.
Death rends his bonds! His prison bursts—un-
loosed!
Behold, audacious King of Terrors comes!
Fiend-form'd and tusk'd—a-gape as Erebus,—
A flame-mouthed Etna in eruption seems!
Arm soul! be strength to meet the Dragon-foe.'

He ceas'd and stood cloud-frowning tenfold Night
That would eclipse the brightest day of Hope—
A dark-wing'd tempest gathering ruin round!

Starless of hope, as whirlwind wheel'd on, up
Grim Death! amock at Hell and scowling at
Despair. From gulf, with Devastation's rush
The Sin-arm'd Curse and all-Devourer storm'd
Impetuous. Night's realms rent at the shock
And felt confusion to her centre Hell.
Awful he stood, vast, horrible and dire
Still howling—'*Blood!*' Wretch'd, cruel, gaunt and grim.
Annihilating Scythe and Life-subduing Dart
Loud-rattling at his side outrageous swung
As livid bolts aleap 'round hand of God.
Locks grizzly, far-down dangling, matted hung
Jaws-famin'd hiding, thro' which baleful eyes
Glar'd dismal—fierce, fell as twin comets look'd
Hell-fir'd and blazing war to nations pale.
His breast still labored! Clouds deep shadow'd thought
Till his distracted mind was skeptic Doubt
That hung him lost as pond'ring Ghost of wo
O'er Ruin's endless tomb—eternal-deep!
Eternity, stood a long solitude,
All thought and darkness and Oblivion—

The still and lone dumb-dead of sepulchres.
One faced he seem'd! and that—infernal Night.
He roll'd eyes wild of utter dreadfulness
And cheek of Darkness deeper death-glares own'd.
His gloom-brows storm-clouds black'ning Chaos
were:
He did not quake! Eyed Death askance and
said,
And all Oblivion trembled as he spake:

'Grim-visaged fiend of frail Mortality!
Down thy world-gorging throat life-blood of Earth
Hath like an ocean vast for centuries pour'd—
Unsatisfied, unfill'd forever-more!
Comest thou to desolate Oblivion?
Then darkness 'stead of feasting thou shalt find
And emptiness and dust in place of blood.
On dust and nothingness canst thou repast?
Will mist and gloom thy burning thirst allay,
Or darkness thy devouring hunger quell?
Then back to Earth;—I give my son's domain:
There slaughter, slay—devour thou and inurn;
But evermore disturb Oblivion not,

Divine her peace and sacred her repose—
Death may not desecrate her quietude.
These Vaults shall ope with Immortality
When God's cloud-coming is the Judgment Morn:
But not Grim Death and Earth and Hell combin'd
With all their forces strong thro' endless years
Could burst Oblivion's adamantine gates
And force from Night her soul-awaiting Dust.
Behold—ETERNITY! her lord and king.
Canst thou O, Fiend! eyelay my dread expanse?
Great Being boundless with her God-crown'd Heavens
To me compared is empty Nothing brought
'Gainst Deity! An ocean shoreless I,—
Space limitless! Duration without end!
Look on me Death, and see thyself—a mite.'

He ended frowning. Indignation dread
From storm-brows leaping, smote, soul-crushingly:—
Chaotic darkness flooding from his face!
With a wide ghostly grin, Death woful stood

By Pestilence, Plague, Famine horror'd round,
And deadly, damn'd as host Infernal seem'd
When thunderstruck to Pandemonium.
Afar, his cave-like jaws down fell, and look'd
Lengths long of ghastliness Starvation-gnaw'd.
He stood a-famin'd! Meager, slim, gaunt, squalid—
All-wretchedness without a parallel!
With a deep dismal gape he shook his bones;
Thro' Desolation's Chambers look'd and howl'd
Apolyon-loud! His baneful eyeballs glare
Lit up dark Dens below! Saw sights, heard sounds
Ne'er saw, ne'er heard before, but saw not—Blood.
Eternity, to groaning statue spake
Down showering Night and scowling Death-despair:

'Behold O, Death! the Dust of other years:
The ghostly Present—Past,—Shades vanish'd all;
The busy brood of antiquated Earth;
Worlds of enigma-wonders wondrous;
Oblivion's own—unheard of evermore;
Dark Ages' waste Tradition can not reach,

And Earthquake-swallow'd Nations from Time's
book
Erased. Volcano-buried cities, towns,
By re-creating Memory forgot.
Mankind from Adam to last son that sleeps.
Eternal mysteries unseen by man,
Beyond the ken of mortal vision far,—
Not Spirit's eye whilst jail'd in flesh and blood—
The swaddling-bands of soul! can bring to
light,
But eye oped only by Eternity.
Behold, Obliv'on's Space-spread bosom void!
Nought's sanctified domain beyond extent,
Where sun comes not to visit Being's pause
Whiles Ages onward roll eternal rounds!
Where Vanity is low, Pride humbled dust—
Worm, Folly, Haughtiness are equals all,
And nought but Virtue towers preeminent.

'How quiet, calm—how lonely and serene
Is the deep sleep of all the hallowed dead
Oned with Oblivion and Forgetfulness!
And those that Fame's oft erring voice applauds.

With these in Memory lock'd, or thron'd within
Affection's heart revered and sacred all,
Alike to dust go down and slumber here,
And nought may save them from Forgetfulness.
Ah! who can fathom the dark gulf of all
The sombre Past, and give to memory
Of Time, the secrets of Eternity
Deep lock'd in chambers of Oblivion?
Oblivion! what greatness moulders in
Thy ghostly hall—unheard of evermore!
Or lives but fable for the Book of Time—
The shadow dim 'mid twilight of Tradition,
All glory gone, and name forgotten long!

'How mountain-high the Dust of Mankind sleeps
The wise the great and good of gone-by years;
Earth's kings, priests, oracles and prodigies—
He—She—It,—all save Spirit of times past!
Earth's cities vast, built by ten million slaves:
Pompeii, Persepolis, Nineveh
With world of life and glory in their walls!
Wrecks wonder'd at these fallen splendors lie
In their death-night inhumed eternally:

They died! and their own hundred-gated walls
Lay round about them ghostly winding sheets;
Their desolations are their sepulchres,
And their own wrecks their monuments and
graves!
Gomorrah Sodom—very hell of Earth!
Jerusalem! the city bright of God
Whose palaces of kings, sky-gilding domes
And battlements bathed in the sunbeam's home,
And God-built temple throned the Deity!
Thebes, Troy, Rome, Balbec, Tyre and Babylon
Abode of heroes and the home of gods—
Sad Desolation's remnants of renown!
In fall a glory and in ruin grand,—
The grandeur of their mighty ruin is
Renown and their eternal epitaph:
Their very dust of former greatness speaks
Till heart sighs out for splendor in the tomb.
And Noah's Ark! and all therein contain'd,
With Raven and her Dove that olive bore,
Which rode sublime and o'er drowned Earth tri-
umph'd,
Have ceased from toil and here serenely rest:—

Sleeps Serpent foul that apple gave to Eve
In sordid night, deceiving now no more.

'King, beggar's dust without reproach, meet here
In soft embrace—all humbleness and love;
Assassin fell and dagger too, harmless
As lambs lie gently mouldering into one,
Nor dream of slaughter, cruelty and blood.
The Hosts of Israel! at sight of whom
Sea fled, to close on Pharaoh's harden'd heart!
By Moses onward led to Promised Land
Where milk and honey in abundance flowed,
Have all left Earth's care-killing woes and pains
For deep Oblivion's peace and quietude.
See OG OF BASHAN! who, on iron bed
Nine cubits long laid ogre-bones to rest.
SAMPSON! that rent in sunder Gaza's posts
Of marble, massy bar and brazen gates,
And hurl'd them high to Hebron's lofty brow.
GOLIAH, too—six cubits and a span!
His iron staff huge as a weaver's beam
He whirled in air while heroes fled away,
And armies of the living God, defied!

Now lies he here the shadow of a shade—
Dust-nothingness one with Oblivion.

'King SOLOMON—God's chosen, Wisdom's crown!
Another name for glory, honor, worth.
Wives, concubines seven and three hundred had,
And horses, servants, chariots—thousands!
Now, Commerce spread her wings at his command,
And with wide Earth's rich stores his coffers
groan'd,—
Made cedars plenteous as sycamore's
Abundance, gold and silver too as stones,
And reign'd e'en over kings—a king of kings!

'Here's one O, Death! for whom thou whetst thy
scythe
Some score of times e'er thou didst make him
thine;
Sure, Time grew weary wasting years on him—
I, jealous, least a rival I beheld!
Oblivion, mock'd, for many centuries groan'd,
And Earth in labor with her burden sigh'd,
E'er his protracted hour had run its course:

But Life's clock struck—"Nine hundred sixty-
nine,"
And Time's bell toll'd a Spirit's flight to Heaven,
When all that was METHUSALAH was mine own—
Rejoicing Darkness bellow'd at the plunge!

'Here Dido, founder of famed Carthage sleeps;
Nimrod of Babylon magnificent;
Cecrops of Athens, Romulus of Rome
And Ashur of imperial Nineveh.
All these, and more, deep in Oblivion lie—
Eternal Mausoleum of Dust and Night!
Where shadow without substance ever sleeps,
And body without spirit rests till morn.
Where Genius—Heaven-lit sun! gives out no
light,
And Homer's harp symphonious doth not sing;
Where Tully's tongue of eloquence is dumb,
The thunder of Demosthenes not heard:
World-ruling Wisdom 's dumb as Chaos-lip,—
Lycurgus, Solon, Plato make no law;
Yea, Priam sleeps unmindful of his Troy,
And Paris mingles with his paramour.

'No Hannibal climbs Alps while trembles Rome;
'Gainst country to conspire no Cataline.
No soul-blind slave to write an Alcoran
Proclaiming loud—'Mahomet is the Christ!'
No frantic monk of Old Enthusiasm
With Murder's mob takes Holy Land by storm.
No Robespierre, Danton and Marat,
Three sulphur flames from deep of Erebus
Alive to Sin and fell Iniquity!
The Satan-sent to work his will on Earth,
To meet Religion meek with Hell's uproar—'

Death in hot haste replied: 'These Hellhounds
fierce
I hiss'd on Man to ruin and destroy!
In robes of Love and Piety and Peace
Wolf Bigotry hath prowl'd wide world around
And gored the heart of e'en God's own Elect
Till Persecution's flames infernal sent
A million Martyrs home to God and Heaven.
These all are gone, but Death 's without his Blood!
Show me thy cells, Oblivion's secret caves:—
Men have escap'd from Earth and my grim jaws

With life,—their blood is in reserve for me.'
Eternity loud replication gave:

'Behold! Oblivion open to thy view—
All Being's blank and Nothing's great extreme
Confusion-pil'd as wrecks of Earthquakes are!
Lo! what gloom-pictures of Departed Joys
Throughout Eternal Chamber mournful hang
Grinning all hideous at wild shriek of Ghosts!
VALE OF FORGETFULNESS opes to thy ken.
Approach. Observe the Shadows of Renown;
The burning meteors of Antiquity;
The living echoes in the ear of Time;
Gigantic Spirits of the Hall of Fame;
Renown'd of Earth—alive by lingering death!
By eye Historic thro' Tradition seen
Dim-dawning in the mist of ancient years,
While blind Doubt cries—'Such Ossians never lived!'
And they, and all but fragments of their works
Housed in the Chambers of Oblivion:—
Names faintly traced on page of Memory,

While Ruin, o'er their former glory lowers
Neglect and nothingness—eternity!

'Dost thou behold the *Poet's* sacred rest?
Heaven's ministers e'er preaching to Posterity!
Boast of their times and fame of ages lived;
The storehouse vast of intellectual sweets,—
Too great a light for Grim Forgetfulness,
And vast a glory for Death-night to hide.
Star-crown on Glory's brow forever-more;
Their living songs do day the world with light—
The light of mind and suns in Time's dark night!
Their laurel crowns outshining far—sceptres
Of gold and diamond coronets of kings:
Their pyramid flames brightest, highest flames
In canopy of Immortality.

'HOMER! whose harp sublime proud Ilium sung,
His name is Glory's ornament and pride!
And Troy embalm'd with immortality.
The first forever in the rolls of Fame—
Fame's wonder and the Muse of Bards for aye,—
The household-god for soul of all the world!

Bright Glory's spire on temple of Renown—
His name is Glory's ornament and pride!
Alone in glory like the sun in heaven
Whose day-bright firmament admits no star:
Terrific rolleth on his thunder-thoughts
And lightnings flash from every lay he sings,—
The Jove of Song! he lives a thunder-peal
In ear of Time till Earth shall be no more.
Odyssea, Iliad! Fame's trumpet blasts
By every Muse divined! The brightest crown
That Immortality and Heaven could give
The sacred brow of their own God-inspired,
To halo with midday Futurity—
The light and wonder of Posterity.

'SAPPHO! crown'd by the tuneful Nine, "Tenth Muse!"
Whose life a poem and fall a drama was.
Her harp Heaven-tuned to sweetest harmony
Eolian, and thoughts a thousand flowers!
The star of Song forever brightest, fix'd,
On diadem of Poesy and Love.
PETRARCH! His harp by Love and Laura strung
Gave him to Fame—the boast of Italy.

'SHAKSPEARE! what diamonds sparkled in thy mind!
A mind-mint coining thought unthought before—
The head and heart of every age for aye!
Reflection's self sat mighty in his soul:
Illumined spirit, Genius unsurpass'd,—
He look'd upon the other side of things!
The child of Nature and the son of Song,—
Inspir'd song peal'd from his immortal harp
As psalm of Heaven by Angel-lyre awoke.
He oped the human heart to eye of man:
His Dramas are Daguerreotypes of Life,
And they map out great Nature like a chart—
Of Nature's own handwriting a fac-simile!
His Works, are a rich rosary of pearls,—
The *fount* of Truth reflecting Passion's soul,
Wherein, the wavy landscape warbling lives,
And many waters with their fishy-stores
Sing, play and dance, or roll foam-crested hills
Confusion-piled and battling with the storm—
By Nereids and all the Tritons loved.
His name, gems wreath of Immortality,—

His broadning fame a mighty tempest sweeps
And roars on ocean-like till Time 's no more.

'MILTON! great teacher of Posterity,
Mind-life and light as Day of Universe.
He oped his lips and words of honey flow'd,
Or Eloquence thunder'd as voice of God.
Singer divine and Angel of the Earth,
He touch'd his lyre and Eden bloom'd again—
More heaven in him than all his age beside!
Immortal Thought's unfathom'd depth sublim'd;
On loftiest wing his towering soul arose
To Wisdom's home and Fancy's Fairy Land
Celestial-plum'd! Then flew to Zion Hill,
Saw Angels, Seraphs saw and Heaven day-gem'd
Sun-radiant with immortal loveliness
Redemption hymning and the Lamb of God
Join'd with the melting melody of spheres,—
One song devout of adoration pure
In living echoes to the Deity.
With Hierarchs convers'd—Jehovah talk'd,
And bask'd in glory of the smile of God!
He lived unknown and unlamented died—

Lived centuries in advance of human kind!
But his prophetic eye saw coming Fame
Ghost-like within the Vale and Shade of Death,
And soul look'd smiles at Immortality!
Too great a light for Death-shades to eclipse
And vast a glory for a tomb to hide:
His name 's on tongue of Praise forever-more—
Sacred to heart of all Posterity.

'BEAUMONT and FLETCHER! Brothers in renown—
Twin-stars in crown of Fame love-wreath'd, soul-wed
Twinkling to eye of Nations yet unborn.
That outcast-noble-beggar see—SAVAGE!
On wretched back hung Poverty all rags—
Want, Hunger's wand awoke his harp to speech!
Remorse, in book of Crime wrote down his name,
But Genius gave him to Posterity,
And Immortality crown'd her inspir'd
With laurel'd victory ever flourishing.

'KIRK WHITE! Poor youth unfortunate! To name

Thy name, Affection's heart drops tears of blood.
His songs are very fragments of his heart,
And speak divinely like an Angel's voice.
Futurity, full oft, with sunny paths
He lit, e'en on to steep of Greatness all
Ascending up, where Glory sits God-like
Alone in vast infinitude of light
High heaven'd on throne of Immortality—
But fell—Fame's own beloved e'er he was twenty!
And Wisdom's sun was death-eclips'd for aye.

'Lord Byron! Honor's own spoil'd son—Love's pet
Hope's child—the heir of Folly and Renown
And wonder wild of loud applauding Earth.
Tho' his life's page is fill'd with Error's blots,
Yet Poesy gave to him the Poet's crown,
And Fame's bright temple high hath own'd him hers—
To shine a star in annals of Futurity
Rich wreath'd with glory ever flourishing.

'In yonder Vale the mighty Heroes sleep
By glorious deeds wed to immortal Fame.

ULYSSES! ardent, bold, wise, eloquent,
The Council's light and valor of the field;
Loud shout of friends and terror of his foes,
A lamb in peace a thunderbolt in storm—
His arm a fortress and himself a host.
Right-nobly born and eminently great,
His glories flamed around him like a sun,—
His history a tale and life a romance!
A galaxy of stars shall crown his brow
And Earth's heart be his living monument.

'ACHILLES! that most terrible of men!
Whose might was armies and whose rage was storm
Fire, death and consternation of the field.
Half god and hero half—invulnerable!
Time-crown'd and sainted in eternity—
By Homer oned with Immortality.
The dreadful breaker of the ranks of war!
Storm-sweeping hero furious as Death!
An Army-routing god—thunderous as Heaven!
Barb'd arrows fell upon him like a rain.
He stood a host, and moveless as a tower
Tho' clouds of spears were tempests in his path,

And legions fear'd his coming and retired.
He came! Bold hearts 'gainst steely-breastplates
leap'd,—
White hung the field pale-shivering in its fear!
He came a god! resistless in his course
Piling a wasteful way with heroes slain.
His falchion lightning, and its fall was deaths,—
Immortals bled—the mighty were in dust,
And fury of his vengeance kill'd remote!

'Beyond all heroes valiant—ALEXANDER!
The prowess of the field, strong arm of fight,
And sharpness of the battle's wasting edge.
Brave, bold and ruinous, with tempest's soul
And thunder's might—fell battle lived in him!
Now, he, from conquering unto conquest swept,
And where he went, went also Fate along,
And Victory advanc'd, or stay'd with him.
His sword's point smote world-enemy around;
Dread heroes stood before him but to fall;
Opposing swords were scatter'd in the dust,
And shields to fragments fell, while Nation's vast
And Kingdoms tumbled to Oblivion.

Unknown to him was fear, or how to fly;
Where danger was, he in his glory stood—
Valor, in Danger's furnace purified!
In storm of arms his soul delighted lived,
And in the battle's shock his brave heart reveled.
Earth was his battle-field, his triumph life,
He lifted up his spear to conquer all—
He met the foe and took them with their spoils!
We name his fields to count his victories.
Like Death, his spirit had a quenchless thirst;
His orphan-breeding sword made desolate;
His hero-felling arm was foe's despair,—
Oppose his might and vanish out of being!
He laid his hand upon the World's great heart
And made it beat in unison with his:
He stamp'd his mark of conquest on mankind,
And they, and their possessions number'd his:—
E'en Earth, bow'd low to his resistless sway
And shouted loud to Fame his name eterne.
Alas! Earth was a unit after all!
And lo! he groan'd for Being's vast domain—
Dropt princely tears to call the stars his own!

'He fell! and Macedonia saw her shroud,
And in his death her own Oblivion:
Worth, wisdom, honor, valor died with him—
Sun sat, and day went out forever-more.
Behold O Death! upon thy arrow's barb
Might lie the greatness all of Alexander
Whom Earth was once too narrow to contain!
That storm of War and Battle's thunderbolt!
The fall of heroes, kingdoms, nations, powers—
World's ashes and the wide spread tomb thereof!

'That ruin, folly of his age—XERXES!
Like Egypt's locust-curse devouring swept,
And led five million men without a head!
Fill'd Greece with troops and seas with vessels fill'd;
Leveled huge mountains that opposed his march—
Drank rivers dry—thought once in all his life,
And wept o'er that as might a silly child!
Look'd on one hundred years to see his hosts
Expire, who did not live so many days!

'E'en merciful when Justice's self cried—'Blood'
Great CESAR was! Name known Creation through,

And wondered at and honor'd far as known,—
That man-of-men of mighty daring made!
He knew not fear and never heard of flight,
The soul of Valor and the battle's life—
The fearful victor of a thousand fields!
World-conqueror—right hand of Victory,—
He hid in Valor's cloak Ambition's deeds.
And who durst stir the kingly lion up?
Great Rome? At "cast of die" the Rubicon
With shout of "*Veni vidi vici*" 's cross'd
And mighty Rome his crown of glory is!
Throne-born, by Valor king'd and all the gods.
The shining wonder 'bove Earth's greatness tow-
er'd—
A living Mars and mortal Jupiter!
War elevated, Peace brighten'd his crest:
Earth's sum of wisdom, virtue, honor, worth,
And light of Rome—her noon without a cloud.
His glory, blazed out blinding to mankind;
Base Envy saw, and sickened at the heaven,—
He fell! and beggard Earth—the world was
wreck—
Imperial Rome lost all in loosing him!

A pyramid of virtue and renown
That lights the skies of Immortality.

'The queen of Egypt—CLEOPATRA see,
Great Cesar's flame and wo of Anthony.
Pomp, Luxury held revels at her court
And table spread with diamonds and with pearls
And ate the wealth of kingdoms at a meal!
Ambition's self was envious to obey
And fleet as hind's foot sped to execute,
While Admiration wild and Wonder gazed,
And brainless Folly rack'd an idiot-brain
For wilds of thought exalted as the heavens
To trumpet forth her worth to panders 'round,
And give with sugar-words and honey-tongue
To Flattery's heart a glorious repast
Of her god-virtues—rivaling all the gods!

'Here, Scotia's hero, greatest of the age—
SIR WILLIAM WALLACE! Victory of Valor.
War-flame in bosom of his patriots—
The heart and soul of every hero's breast!
His strong arm's valor was his country's hope,—

What buckler stayed the falling of his sword?
His claymore's edge was fate, fall many deaths;
Piled wide around him lay the mountain-slain—
Victorious ever and forever great.
He, in the greatness of his glory towered—
Outpouring of his strength was majesty;
Wond'rous to men the story of his might
All greatness save great Wallace' self excelling.
Proud England saw the hero and she quak'd;
Her thousands met his little band and fell.
He came! chains of Oppression pinch'd no more;
Slavery went free; Hope, Happiness look'd smiles
At Freedom,—Liberty had resurrection!
He was his country's bulwark and defence,
Her peace, her savior—Scotia lived in him!
His monument is—Freedom, Liberty,
And wisdom, justice, valor, virtue, worth,
Halo with heaven his immortality.
He was betrayed to make all ages mourn;
One Earth-wide tear his hapless fall embalms—
All think of his death-butchery to weep.
He lies a martyr envied in his tomb,—
His fall on Edward's name stamp'd—'Infamy.'

'See Valor's own and Wisdom's—BONAPARTE!
The bravest, he, where all around were brave,
The mighty terror of a thousand fields,—
Poesy-sung and all alive to fame.
Kind Fortune's smile to throne imperial clumb
And sat thereon like a divinity,—
A throne self-built upon heroic dust.
All-glorious thinner of the ranks of war!
His feats death-daring, Envy loves to lisp,
And foes, dumb, pale, all sanction them around.
Soul of the age and body of the times;
The lion-hearted, toil-enduring chief—
Surge-repelling rock 'mid Ocean's billows!
Swords could not reach, nor cannons lay him low.
He came Heaven's thunderbolt, and ruin was,—
The battle's strength, and Vengeance dwelt with him.
A world-consuming comet of a man!
His march shook continents and smote nations;
His rush upon the foe was terrible,—
His cannons, earthquakes were to isles remote!
With mountain-dead, red Carnage pil'd the plain,

And blood-paths stream'd thro' world-wide enemy—
A Desolation sweeping desolate!

'Here, Moralists, and there the Statesmen sleep:—
George Washington! Earth's pride and more than king—
Heaven's chosen sent to set a Nation free—
Columbia, thee—Eden of Liberty!
His world-wide throne the heart of all mankind.
Beloved of Freedom and the bless'd of Heaven,—
He was of sacred Freedom born, and drank
In Liberty with his own mother's milk—
His cradle-song the song of Liberty!
Renown of arms and ornament of Peace!
His country's savior and that country's love;
Lyre's voice, and odes of many cannons' mouths.
Great parallel to Piety and Worth;
Just, noble, brave—hero to God and man,—
One whom Religion's self delights to laud!
His righteous steps attendant Angels led;
Safety and Honor walk'd with him along—
Espous'd of Wisdom and beloved of Heaven!
Heaven's own anointed and her God-inspired

Divinity of greatness, glory of renown!
His greatness, would with Glory's light halo
All-lustrous, diadem of Universe,
And virtue, to its throne add ornament:—
One whom e'en Envy's tongue calls good and wise.
He stood with Virtue—kings were humbled;
He met vast armies—they were scatter'd all;
He for Columbia pray'd, and Victory came,
And Freedom from Oppression leap'd and lived.
His wonderous deeds exalteth Heroism,
And Honor's path 's illumin'd with his god-light.
Like his great Parent—God! he gave to men
Treasure divine, e'en—FREEDOM—LIBERTY,
And INDEPENDENCE crown'd Columbia's brow!

'His people's father fell—the full of years!
Death laid all but his virtues in the dust—
The noblest ashes that enriches urn!
Love-tears wide-streaming from a Nation's heart
Pour'd sacred to immortal Washington.
The tomb's embalm'd with glory where he rests;
He lives revered by an admiring world.
His glory, may not know Oblivion,

Nor fame, the blight of Old Antiquity;
Renown, shall ever proudly ring his name
To vast Futurity delighted, loved.
Let Heaven's bright sun grow dim and be blown
out,
But Virtue's own adorned can never fade—
They blaze and sparkle one eternal day.

'In knowledge great and in all goodness full
See NEWTON,—mirror of intelligence!
Sage Reason on his heart exalted sat,
And kindled in his breast celestial fires.
With Contemplation's self he soar'd aloft
Thro' Nature's bounds and Being's mighty maze—
Unveil'd the handiwork of Deity,
And gazing on its loveliness was charm'd.
His wisdom-fill'd and soul-illumin'd mind
Gave Science heaven, and call'd Starland his own,
And named the gems Night's diadem adorning.
He deeply drank from Learning's magic cup
The food celestial of immortal Truth,
And by his intellect God-luminous
Old Mystery's vast abode of darkness lit

As Spirit at Creation "water's face,"
And countless Worlds from void leap'd into life
And light reveal'd, and gave their names to man.
High Honor, glorifies his brow with stars:
In orb of his own immortality
He sweeps a sun in Wisdom's firmament
Brightning to eye of all posterity.
And by his side—sage of America!
The thunderous and majestic FRANKLIN lies
In his own Lightning's fiery terrors clad—
The Jove-arm'd master of the bolts of Heaven!
He look'd thro' Nature with a Poet's eye;
He tam'd the Thunder-bolt as hand of God,
And made fork'd Lightning—servant of mankind!
The world is wiser by his living in't.
Immortal Wisdom's crown and Freedom's star—
The son beloved of glorious Patriotism!
He lives forever in the halls of Fame,—
His fame shall mock at bald Antiquity
And shine all lustrous when Time's self 's no more.

'Behold O, Death—VALE OF ELYSIUM!
Where Peace and Love in sacred slumber sleep,

And Virtue is embalm'd in smile of Heaven.
Bower once of Happiness, garden of God
Where Adam dwelt heart-wed, one with his Eve—
Heaven's Beauty blooming Eden-loveliness!
Eden! by swords of God's Arch-angels kept
Till Earthquake hurl'd it to Eternity,
And the Earth-heaven was deep Oblivion!
Its empty name, alone, shall ever live
A sacred echo in the ear of Time—
A wonder-mystery for the trump of Fame!
Not Poesy divine with harp inspired,
To Earth shall Eden give—her fairy hand
Can never pluck it from Oblivion.

'Lo, here great HOWARD sleeps! whose saint-like deeds
Of charity, bade Sickness send full soul
Of praise devout to Heaven for Gilead's balm,
While bless'd Benevolence loud rang the name
And works and worth of her own son beloved
Down to Posterity—hallowed by all.
The crown'd of Virtue and the loved of God!
To noblest deeds and labours sweet of love

His towering soul of sympathy aspired,
And oned him with well-being of a world:
His arms of charity compassion-spread
Were ocean-like—embracing all mankind.
He rear'd his fame by happiness of man;
He laid the World's vast wretchedness full stretch'd
Groaning and bleeding on a naked heart,
And his Earth-wide humanity down shower'd
Water of life for every mortal wound,
And found there is a heaven in being good.
Friend of the friendless—glory of his kind,—
Loved Mercy's Angel ever on the wing!
He came, and with him, also, bless'd Relief,
Wide strewing joy, as the bright sun the day,
And made the heart of Gratitude his own:
His wide-oped hand shower'd charities afar,
While Poverty smil'd blessings where he came
And hail'd her kind preserver as he passed.
Lived not for self but for the good of all,—
There was a world-soul in this Heaven-sent man
All livingly alive to wants of Earth—
Heart-full of love to God and to mankind:
He, peace to Trouble, comfort unto Grief

And clothes to naked, feasts to Famine gave—
Starvation, Sorrow, Suffering saw the good
Samaritan, and leap'd for joy and lived,
While lip of Mourning blossom'd into smiles.
His gifts, were all a healing balm to Wo,
And laughing plenty to the cot of Want
That bade the flash of bliss from all eyes leap:
His works of worth were numberless to man,—
They fill a page in the great Book of Life
Imperishable as his eternity.
His heaven-illumin'd dust divinely glows
With Glory's light all lustrous as a sun;
His virtues scatter many stars around,
Whose constellations diamond his renown
And day his immortality for aye.
Admiring Nations loud applaud the saint;
Great souls sigh out for virtuous fame like his,—
His growing fame will rend the brazen doors
To very heart of base Ingratitude,
And Howard's name, e'en in that satan-home
Shall reign revered, exalted and alone—
One more than mortal and just less than God.

'In Horror's Vale and Shadow of grim Night
Lo—GULF OF SIN! embosomed in Despair.
Dread world of Sorrow dismal and forlorn
As Death-jaws—spirit-loosing, ruinous!
Shade Valley of Old Chaos and of Hell
Where utter Darkness is imbodied dense;
Where Ghosts forever shriek hideous and dire,
And pallid Fear, Remorse, Affright wild eyed
And wrinkled Grief and Wretchedness and Wo
With Fiends infernal and with Demons curs'd
Breathe sulphur flame and roar out blasphemies
In devil-hate—all-damn'd as Erebus.
The Wicked sleep abandon'd here by Hope:
Betrayer of great Wallace see—MONTEITH!
Like a huge blot on brow hangs—Infamy.
Contempt and biting Scorn with serpent tongues
Shall hiss the wretch down to Posterity
A shame, a curse, a Judas and—devil!

'Here, too, lies GINGHAS KHAN and TAMERLANE—
Madmen! who made their realms the slaughter-house
Of Tyranny, Crime, Inhumanity,
And drain'd life-floods from heart of Innocence

To wreathe their murd'rous brows with infamy,
And croak their hateful names despised as Sin
To haggard ear of everlasting Hate
Fame-damn'd to a curs'd immortality—
Fell monsters shunn'd beyond the name of Hell.

'NERO! Renown'd for folly and for vice!
Another name for bloody Murder, fool
Wretch, Cruelty and base Brutality—
All the Ten Plagues of Egypt in one man!
The fen of Nonsense, sink of Vanity
By curses of mankind immortal made.
All sordid dust and night behold he lies,
Nor burns great Rome, nor his own mother slays!
How oft have low-born Immorality
And cloven-footed satan Tyranny,
Sat throne of kings and sceptres sway'd to scourge
The world, and by the hatred of mankind!
He, devil-hearted Persecution brought
From her low-deep, and Torture's dragon-claw
Gored Zion sore for centuries to come.
Upon his life's whole page he stamp'd—Foolery
Of Hell and demon crime, that Earth might see—

A fool's misdeeds are history of Crime.
Dethron'd he died: Imperial Rome had one
Destroyer less, and Hell one victim more.
His fame 's a blot on temple of Renown;—
His bloody name with his life-deeds accursed,
Are thought of e'er to make the good man weep.

'More monster than a man he lived, and turn'd
When dead to monster quite, huge MAXIMIN!
To rival the vile brute strove hard—excell'd,—
To infamy on through the paths of Shame!
By swine-like gluttony and by beast-strength
To temple clumb of Immortality—
The laugh and scoff of all posterity.
Behold O, Death! deep in dark Vaults below,
Ten thousand more vain idiots that proved
By demonstration clear, that Satan in
Them dwelt—his workshop forging out his will!
And many pass'd Accountability
And into witches vile, or wizzards turn'd,
While bellow'd Hell and Legion mark'd her own.
Here, direful Shadows of departed power,
And mortal-satans wedded to the Shades!

The greedy Earth their gory foot-prints drank;
Their names and deeds are with Forgetfulness—
Oblivion's grim Spectres of the Past!'

He ceas'd to speak to Death. Majestic stood.
His look, Night-clouds that flood from Den of Wo—
Chaotic Darkness storming from his face!
Two-fac'd he seem'd! this one, the horrors fell
Of Horror told, and that smile-lit gleam'd Heaven.
Same time, to all the Righteous sweetly spake,
And roar'd to Sin as thunderbolts of God!
Awe was. Fire-eyes lit all Oblivion round.
Death silent stood. His eye roll'd bloody-wilds
Wild-staring as Affright grinning at Hell—
Astonishment soul quaking at the sight!
His combin'd locks like adder's deadly folds
Half hid his goblin cheek by Famine coil'd—
Death-agony fierce-scowling at Despair!

Eternity smote Darkness with his wand!
He, and Grim Death down sank to *Nameless Night*
Where Silence Chambers spread without a bound
And Chaos reigns o'er blank Forgetfulness
Annihilation and Eternal Death.

BOOK IV.

The Closing Scene.

BOOK IV.

On holy Vision's heavenly wing upborne,
Thro' Nonexistence' vast domain I flew
Swift as the meteor of a cloudless sky
To Silence Halls in Vale of Nameless Night
Where roar Eternal thunder'd thus to Death:

'Thou life-devouring Dragon arm'd by Sin,
Behold Jehovah's heaven before Heaven was!
Confusion's reign and Emptiness supreme
Where Order 's not and Being hath no name.
A shoreless void by Spirit unillumed—
Eternal Blackness blinding and alone

Without a light to make it visible!
A shapeless wild of wonder and amaze
Where Nothingness reigns soulless and upright,
And Silence lives without a voice, or tongue,—
Old Silence Den and Mystery for aye
Lowering forever at Nonentity!
Existence-lifeless, Vacuum infinite—
Infinitude of Emptiness and Nought,
And Imperfection perfect and complete.
Chaotic darkness without form and void,
Creations uncreate—too dumb, deaf, dead
To hear the great Creator's voice proclaim
To moving Chaos' all affrighten'd ear:
'Existence! forth from Nonexistence come.'
Many a lifeless Heaven in embryo!
Nonentity that hath not look'd on God!
Blank Nothing's shadow and Eternal Night's!

'Here, *Fame's Forgotten* sleep—Oblivion's own!
Unknown to Echo is their home secure.
Forgetfulness, erased from Book of Time
Their names with all their deeds, and hurl'd them
forth

Fame's lost—Oblivion's oned forever-more.
Dreams talk not with these Shades departed long,
Night-visions speak not of their memories.
Here, Old Antiquity, once throned with Fame
And crown'd with wonder and the World's applause,
With all her Time-forgotten Cities sleep.
Behold! Antediluv'an Idols all,
With Myst'ries numberless of Eld renown'd
From Memory's mighty volume long erased
And from the annals vast of Ages gone
By dreadful besom of Destruction swept,
All lost in Night and Grim Forgetfulness—
Oblivion-shadows and eternity!

'Lo! here is one who tower'd on earth Fame's own:
His statues grew beneath his plastic hand;
His chisel'd magic was the marble's glow;
He touch'd the rock,—it stood erect and lived—
A Fairy-wonder and a speaking art!
Creator-like, to Chaos said—'Come forth:'
Beauty arose from dust and being had,—
Dumb marble heard! life, love came from cold stone,
And into Angels turn'd, some into—gods!

Each form divine was Genius' self reveal'd,
And every feature Poesy enthron'd
Whose life-looks spake immortal finger's touch!
The soul-inspired image gave he breath,
From new-creation spirit look'd and—talk'd!
Perfection, smiling, call'd the work her own.
Now lies he here, and wed to Nameless Night;
His name and genius are—Oblivion:
His glory's works and age in which he lived,
The heaven-oped eye of Wisdom cannot reach.

'Here sleeps IMAGINATION'S fairy child!
Bright Fancy's loved and Inspiration's own,
Who made great Nature but his dwelling place
And took Creation captive at his will.
He had his home upon an Angel's wing,
And sped from Light's full fount to Darkness depth
Swift as the soul from prison door of frail
Mortality, to gate of Paradise.
Soul's eye was ope! and while yet dungeon'd deep
In flesh, it pierc'd the present, future, past
Scanning all mysteries there in embryo,
And then reveal'd a marvel to mankind.

Great Being's self he bounded at a glance,
And folded up Existence in a thought;
Then took sublime his awful plunge profound
To lowest deep! Scan'd desolation fell
And wo and death and ruin manifold
That down forever with the weight of worlds
On dread Apolyon's brow pour thundering.
With bottomless abyss, his soul mingled!
Hung long on dismal wail of black Despair—
Was oned and lost with the infernal howl
And hideous shriek of Wo-gnaw'd Spirits damn'd!
Thence soar'd at will thro' mighty Void of
    Space—
With Angels winged the sacred Mount of God
And bands Seraphic saw—saw the Redeem'd
And bask'd in the sun-smile of Deity,
Till deep immersed with Inspiration's fire
He burning sped with glory's sacred flame
To atmosphere poor fallen Earth with Heaven,
And give mortality an immortality.
But Satan dwelling in one foolish Omer,
The library burn'd that treasured all his works,
And he is mine—dust and Oblivion.

'Behold the dust whose soul was ELOQUENCE!
He stood man's friend and the beloved of God—
Embodied Wisdom chasing Ignorance.
His tongue was potent, and well train'd to speak
The God-inspired language of the heart
In Passion's own divinity of tongues;
His voice Heaven-tuned to native harmonies—
A sweeter sound young Zephyr breath'd;
His thoughts were revelations of the Truth
Array'd in Beauty's garb—sparkling indeed!
He painted pictures as great Nature doth,
And on the soul they rush'd subduingly.
From well-bent bow of his own giant mind
Darts of Conviction and Conversion sped
Celestial-barb'd to centre of the mark,
Whiles Folly felt the death and fell, or flew,—
Heart-pathos reaching to the fount of tears!
His every gesture had the powers of speech,
Orations many spake in speaking one—
The fires divine bright beaming from his eye
Soul-eloquence to Nature thundering!
Each feature, look was passion, dignity;
Each move pow'r, action—Nature breath'd in all.

He spake! the hearts of all his hearers fill'd,
And souls afar from their celestial homes
Drank saving wisdom from the fount of Light
To chase the cloud from Life's drear pilgrimage
And smooth the path to their own native Heaven.
All common-place he left to little men,
And soar'd at will infinitude of space
Thro' starry flights original and grand
Where Glory dwells with her beatitudes
Illumined by light of the Eternal Day.
With mild Persuasion's magic wand he took
Earth spell-bound—hung the world upon his lip!
Was Reason's self detecting fallacies,
And Logic's wand and death of Sophistry:
He weigh'd the truth on scales of Certitude,
When Truth came forth as orient as Morn
Firing the void of dun Obscurity,
And day from night as Earth from Chaos rose
And chased all fog, mist, gloom as evil dreams
Till Demonstration flam'd from face of Argument
And Reason stood reveal'd—Omnipotent.

'He knew to thunder well in Passion's storm:

On love, soft as the breathings of the lute,
Against Crime crushing as an avalanche.
He spake, and awed—Nations! The people all
With wonder wild, loud shouted him applause:
He spake to soul! it trembled at the shock
And Spirit leap'd as tho' a god had spoken.
His every word, look, tone, all—Oracle!
They lived, breath'd, burn'd and spake to near and
far:
'Behold! a soul sublimed and Angel-winged
Amid the starry heavens speeding at will
Fire-char'ot of soul-loosing Eloquence!'
In speeches, all, revolved both life and death,
And nought save Virtue could withstand the shock
And face the power of his oratory.
His argument swept dreadful as the storm,
And holy fires out-flashing near and far
Down fell wide-wasting as the thunderbolt—
Ruin was! Blind Error died a thousand deaths,
Doubt fled, Sin fell, whiles Certainty stood firm.

'He was a library vast by Wisdom fill'd
With knowledge teeming o'er, and giant thoughts

Like mountains rolled within his sea-like mind
'Bove man to tell; and oft-times with closed lip
Stood Spirit-voiced and thundering like a god!
Fire-tongues that spake were in that *pause* divine—
Heart-passion lightning from his speaking face,—
All soul-sublimity allied to Heaven!
Lost hearts enraptured kindled at the flame,
And God-fill'd spirits sup'd with Deity.

'Here 's one O, Death! who while he lived on Earth,
Had heart of fiend and soul of hell, that spake
A devil quite! His lying tongue was like
The viper's—fork'd! and deadly venom dropp'd.
His midnight-mind was baneful Envy's home
Where SLANDER sat enthroned 'bove name of God.
Upon his lip hung fetid poison—green!
The adder's tongue was harmless by its side
And innocent her sting with his compar'd—
A name diseas'd what medicine can heal?
Dishonor is life's grave that swallows down
Alive its prey that no redemption knows.
His cloven foot trod sacred names in dust,
And his delight to ruin was, devour,—

Strove to dishonor all the works of God!
To number neighbors-faults his chief employ,
And lo! the sum complete told not his own!
In Virtue's Eden, Satan-like he leap'd,
Peace, Honor, Reputation, Character
Bled at each pore, while his satanic soul
Rejoic'd aloud o'er Holiness debas'd,
Good name in jaws of Infamy and Death—
Death crown'd with triumph, grave with victory!
He lived to bark at Glory and Renown,
And dog both Worth and Virtue to the tomb:
He followed Merit howling as he went—
Calumnies shot to Reputation's dome,
And glory sought in pulling Glory down—
For Greatness, groan'd, while seeking to defame!

'See one, whose life was but a waning moon,
Himself an ocean smote by every breeze,—
A fickle sea forever troubled, toss'd
To foam,—lash'd by each idle wind that blew!
Chameleon-like he was—green, red, white, black
All in the compass of one little hour.
Had his face changed as his inconstant mind

His own wretch'd mother had not known her child.
He was a sick-man's pulse and Winter's cold
And Summer's heat at once—true but to change!
He loved to day heart's hate of yesterday,
Then loathed as soon each thing he ever loved.
His ways were all like breath on face of steel
Soon on, soon off; or blush of Modesty
Red—pale as quick, and fluctuating still :—
Was true to nothing but to FICKLENESS,
And constant only in inconstancy!

'Here sleeps Heaven's own, her chosen and inspired—
Her Song-anointed Angel of the Earth
Who gave harp speech as the bright ones above!
The Muse of Earth and POET of all times,
The flight of Spirit and the wing of Mind—
One born to soar as eagle to the skies!
His fancy was as rosy morning's smile,
Imagination as a mid-day sun;
He had a mind that grasps the infinite
And brought to light unfathom'd mysteries.
The hill of Difficulty clumb alone,

Unaided to the steep of Greatness hied
As to his home. With Fame walk'd hand in hand—
Convers'd familiar as a friend with friend.

'Wisdom and Virtue's own—the mild and pure!
While in the world, he lived above it far—
A passer-by to all but soul of things:
So little earth was in this man of men,
Her witch-like charms led not his heart astray;
His spirit scorned to be bond-slave of Earth—
The drudge of dust and bauble of a minute!
His muse-exalted soul was e'er on wing
A-soar for Immortality and God,
And his cup's fullness ecstacy and heaven.
Bright Fancy's child 'lone equal'd by a god!
Inspir'd, and all too like the Angel-ones
To be enchanted with the prose of things—
Too Fairy-like to mix ethereal being
With dust-like dullness of slave-driving Earth
Sin-fill'd with inhumanity and death.
His life one beauteous vision was of Heaven,
His whole existence warble of a bird—
One melody—the every Muse of Song!

'He dwelt from earth apart with Solitude
Where boundless Nature was his all in all,
Mused where the widowed turtle loved to mourn
And Poesy tower'd sublime with laurel'd head,
Abiding there a heaven-sent hermit lone
Of rocks and caves and Nature and the Muse!
And Eden was where e'er his footsteps strayed
For all within was Paradise and Peace.
With inspiration brightning into day
He on a rude cliff's height that ruin frown'd
To a wild-howling gulf beneath, sat wrapt,
Dark Mystery's inmost chambers searching all,—
Nature unveil'd—admired her nakedness!

'With Seraph's zeal and holy rapture fired
He struck his lyre and gave his soul to Song—
Eye kindling as Poetic Vision rose:
He sang! the charm of sound was heard afar
Loud pealing hymns of greatness unto God;
Great thoughts like fires celestial sparkled bright,
And scenes unseen before and flesh from Heaven
As Etna blazed and dazzled lands remote.
He sped at will thro' Fairy Land, upon

Bless'd Fancy's wing flew Heaven—the clouds and storms
Beneath his feet and God alone above!
He soar'd at home to Light's remotest smile,
Drank spirit-scenes from Glory's highest tower;
Or sank amid Chaotic-wonders lost
E'er God-lit Being throned a Deity!
And view'd at will Creation's mighty wild
A sleepless void of dreamless nothingness;
Hell flameless, and yon Heaven a shadow all;
Angels and Seraphim but golden dust,
And Immortality's sun unillumed,—
Found nought but dread Omnipotence alone!
He hunger'd after glorious flights, and soul
Thirsted to bask in sacred Fount of Song
And write with Inspiration's holy pen
Dipped in the dew of Fame divine, his name
Highest on spire of Immortality.

'He classic made the home in which he lived
And sacred every sod his footsteps press'd;
Yea, his lyre's magic resurrection was
To dust in vaults of Old Antiquity—

Being to bosom of Oblivion!
Things buried long forth from their graves arose,
And life and beauty gave to breathless forms—
To very stones and senseless rocks lent tongues!
From womb of Mystery new creations leap'd;
The home of Darkness glorious Light illumined,
And man lived centuries with Futurity!

'Fame's trumpet huge fill'd with his glorious name
Till Envy wept and sighed herself away,—
World-famous! Praise surrounded him as light:
He wrapt high Honor 'round him like a robe—
Wrestled with Glory's self and made her his!
Posterity his debtor is:—she pays
Him not! He died and is forgotten quite.
Dark ages long this sun of Fame eclipsed;
The vale of Nameless Night treasures his dust,
Forgetfulness his glory and his name.
So let him rest in arms of Quietude
Till Judgment Morn with thunders shall awake
The tomb to noon with present Deity,
And then the Poet shall arise and burn

A God-illumined Spirit of pure light—
Bright Glory's own, day-flaming like a sun.

'Lo! here is one, who while he was on Earth,
With Contemplation deep, secluded lived
In moss-grown dwelling of ancestral fame,
And up to mountain-home of WISDOM walk'd
To pluck bright Knowledge from her hidden depth
And revel in the heart of Mystery:—
Deep thoughted Wisdom's giant tower of mind!
Full oft he sat with Contemplation's self
Deep musing long in a wild cave retired,
The busy world shut out, and nought was found
Save soul up-reaching—on, to find its God.
He loved converse with self, loved silence much
And sweet retirement and lone solitude:—
Less idle ne'er than when he idle was,
And never less alone than when alone.
Desired to hear, more than he sought to speak,
For he was bless'd with one less tongue than ears:
He wore a seal upon his clos'd-up lips,
And ever loved to think, while Folly talk'd.
Knew what, when, where to speak to purpose true—

Effect, and also to keep silence knew:
Speech e'er unbar'd his lips and heart at once,
While very soul rode forth with Eloquence.
His wisdom's fire like sun to morning, light
To darkness gave, and sombre Ignorance
Beheld the flame in her chaotic home.
When lean'd his brow on hand, his laboring soul
From thoughtfulness profound, brought wonders forth,
And mysteries mysterious unveiled
Marv'lous to eye of all futurity:
Mid Doubt's gloom-wilderness mid-day sprang up,
And Knowledge rose and smil'd at Certainty.
His mighty mind sat mirror'd in his look;
His spirit-speaking face reveal'd a soul
Where image of a God was visible,
And handiwork of great Omnipotence:
Intensity of thought his sage brow crown'd,—
Forth from his eye the very lightnings leap'd,
And men look'd reverence at him as he pass'd.

'He tower'd aloft a miracle of mind,
A mount of light illuming to the world—

A blazing sun in Wisdom's firmament!
By Genius' fire and flame of Science' torch
The womb of dark Obscurity he lit
And Knowledge' self revealed her ways to man;
On Learning's wing he upward sped star-high,
And number'd o'er and named each diamond orb
On Night's bespangled bosom burning bright.
His all-subduing thought thro' Mystery drove
Wedge-like! He saw in darkness, and as light
Immortal was, for midday dwelt with him:—
Unfolded Nature as a book, and read
At will to man—the manuscript of Heaven.
World-light! Around him thronging Nation's
flock'd;
They, basking in his sunbeams found the day—
Feasting on manna and the bread of life,
Till death-eclips'd by darkness and the tomb
Was Wisdom's sun—and all the world was night.

'Here 's one, who while he lived thought little
thoughts,
Spake much, and ever spake before he thought—
Loud rattling many nothings in an hour!

His fluency of tongue without the oil
Of Wisdom ran, and demonstrations gave
To all—of mind's machinery out of tune:
In him had silence been Wisdom's sublime.
His woful want of intellect, wrote—'FOOL'
Upon his soulless face in capitals.
He never read a book, or saw himself,
Yet thought poor self the greatest man alive!
So little knew he sought to know no more—
Was e'en too dull to learn in school of sage
Experience—the alphabet of things!
His head was fill'd with Folly's maze of mist;
In chamber dark of Ignorance soul slept,
And brute alone and dust were visible.
What weight of ignorance, stupidity—
What depths of darkness and of nothingness,
And what profundity of nonsense all
Were in that little, mole-like head of his
Unknown to sense and hollow as a gourd!
Sense stood agape at his stupidity
Till Feeling's heart bled inward, and she wept,
And Pity, from tear-loaded heart sigh'd out:
'A world-jest! Wonder winning every eye

E'en Folly's shadow of the Fall of Man!
Creation yet in her chaotic state!
Dawn dimly faint of an immortal soul!
Jehovah's image shrouded deep in death—
Eternal likeness buried in the dust!'

'The HYPOCRITE,—deception eloquent!
Who wore a double tongue new-oiled and smooth
Glib, voluble—a well-dissembl'd sin!
Chameleonized she every color wore
That Nature owns—a rainbow of all dies!
Her soul was dragon-mazes of Deceit
Wherein Destruction's daggers were conceal'd;
Her mouth was Falsehood's home and house of
Guile,
Envenomed breath the bane of Perfidy:
Her words were treachery; her love was hate;
Her smiles so many deaths all dragon-arm'd;
Her kisses death-masks and vile serpent charms,
And her embrace the dagger's deadly stab;—
Beguiling, wooing, charming to betray,
And cheat self more than all the world beside!
Loath'd crocodile—e'er weeping to devour!

A lip-deluding, heart-concealing death!
Vile contradiction and a living lie!

'The Devil's fool she was in Virtue's garb
With hell in thoughts by scripture honeyed all—
God on her lips and Legion at her heart!
A seeming christian while a very fiend—
Fattening for day of dreadful slaughter near
And ripening for the fire—ne'er to be quench'd!
The laugh of fiends by God and man despised.
In holy armor clad she fought for Sin—
Wrestling with God to gain applause of men!
Besieging Heaven to take by storm—a purse!
Her adoration-lifted hand grasp'd Earth!
Fell wolf in sheepfold of the Lord of Life!
Wash'd wickedness baptised to fouler stains!
She, half a Satan was, e'er Satan's own.

'Here 's one who look'd a yawn and lived a dream!
His walk claimed kindred with the torpid sloath,
And his stupidity with doltish jack,—
His sluggish pace the lip to laughter moved!
His gluttony and gruntings were the hog's,

And growlings, snarlings, snappings as the dog's,
While lo! his form erect, shadow'd—a man!
He pass'd Care careless by, and heedless grinn'd;
His days he spent in sleep, nights in debauch;
He when not hungry ate—drank tho' not dry,
And when he needed no repose he slept.
He only lived to eat, to drink, to sleep
And pull his raiment off and put it on—
Hot hasting down to poverty and shame,
And ever in Temptation's road to Sin
And death and hell—tempting the Tempter stood!
He was an unbent bow unfit for use,
A lounger in the home of INDOLENCE,
A foe to health of body, peace of mind.
His torpid body sottish and relaxed,
Invited Pestilence to house with him—
World-cipher and the murderer of time!
Desires were all asleep and senses dead;
Life was a living death and time a waste;
He was the grave of life entombing soul
That feign would be on wing to find its God—
Live-corpse, by Idleness inhum'd alive!
Blank of existence and life-chaos he—

Life-vacuum abhorr'd by Nature's self!
He ever rested without lassitude,
Sought to be idle, to do nothing strove,
Sweet rest to him a heavy labor was—
Fatigued to death with having nought to do!
He to no purpose lived, and died—not miss'd,
Bequeathing to his wretch'd posterity—
Dishonor, ignorance and poverty.

'See one who wore a shallow mind and heart
Corrupt upon her back, that passers-by
Her folly might behold! She spent her all
(And not to please her own, but other's eyes,)
Her body to adorn and soul forget!
Life's chase was after Vanity and Vice;
A dangling curl hid God from view, and toys
Out weigh'd Heaven and eternity of bliss.
Walked FASHION's rounds of haughtiness and sin,
In the straight-jacket of Politeness dress'd
Priding in peacock-splendors of her short
Liv'd rags—fig-leaf array of fallen Earth!
While brainless Folly mark'd her dear beloved.
She hung her happiness on Flattery's lip;

Her peace upon the whisper of Applause;
Her joy one look of praise; a bow, a nod
Was heaven enough, and fill'd each vain desire.
One solemn thought of winding-sheet, or Hell,
Was life's eclipse that horrified the soul,
Or thought on death—perdition to her peace.
In self she dared not look, for nought was there
Save Foolery and Old Man with his deeds:—
Beyond the grave? Despair stood hideous there
Eclipsing every hope! therefore balls, plays
And parties thickly crowded 'round her heart
Beguiling wo with Siren smile of peace.
Earth was her Heaven and her eternal all—
Her hope, desire and every wish she had:
She knew not self, and flew from Wisdom's light
And scorn'd to taste a Savior's pardoning love.
Ofttimes she stood for hours 'twixt comb and glass—
A painting at a gaudy image gazed!
While Judgement's councils sat on every hair
She curl'd, and one amiss high treason deem'd
'Gainst common wealth of Vanity and Sin.
A wrinkle gave affright; a hair turn'd gray
A dread assassin seem'd, destroying all

Her bliss, and soon as seen—pluck'd out wild-eyed!
Her heart was home of Fickleness and death,
And soul the throne of Arrogance and Pride—
So little soul within that she was vain!
With Folly's self thro' Fashion's giddy rounds
Light trip'd the gaudy toy e'er rustling on
Wide way along in her unpaid-for silks!
A guilded-sorrow, white-wash'd wretchedness,—
Creation's bastard, blushing painted grace!
Vain Fashion is base Folly's willing slave
Whom paint can't turn to loveliness and charms.

'A butterfly existence thus she lived
A-flitting onward thro' vacuity
Of life, to blind with tinsel show the gaze
Of her own brother worms! And night and day
She strove with labor, cost and agony
Ridiculousness to sublime, and take
By storm of hypocritic subtlety
A coxcomb's heart as empty as her own!

'Here lies the pride of old Antiquity:
Creation was in magic of his art—

Life, light and shade oblivious mingling!
The very breath of life was to be seen
In pictures' look that talk'd of intellect!
A speaking image rose from pencil's touch
At will, and to beholders cried aloud:
'Here, Art and Nature you behold on strife;
Perfection's self stands heaping doubt on doubt
Long lost whiles judging which hath mastery.'
His living canvass was Life's mirror true,
Where goddess Nature looking day by day
Saw her heaven-face reflecting Deity:
Ay, he could paint the antic wilds, and arch
Shrewd meaning of the monkey's eye! He touch'd
Young Beauty's cheeks and poetized her charms,
While Angel-beauties smil'd them into life!
Each form did voice itself and fasten 'round
The heart, and features all look'd spirit forth
And inspiration wed to Immortality.
But now with Grim Forgetfulness he lies
Night's nameless one eternized with Oblivion.

'All these have given their riches up and power
Ambition, greatness, wisdom, folly, fame—

Lost, oned with Gulf of Darkness all profound.
But drop of blood in all canst thou behold?
Who seeketh blood within Oblivion's realms
Of ruin, dust and night shall seek in vain:—
Haste! I give Earth and all therein contained;
Her mighty ruler, too, I give—her king
Oblivion's runaway—mine only son!
Who, from deep hollow of my side eloped
To Being's God-lit throne and call'd him—
TIME.
Ah, haste thee Death! to conquest now arouse
And be a storm,—to desolation sweep
And war thy might for blood where blood is
found:—
O! rend, slay, kill, consume, blast and devour
Each thing that lives, moves, breathes and grows
within
The hollow of Almighty Maker's heaven
Expanded hand that ruleth over all
And all directs. Blast Time's fleet-flying wing—
Existence-ruling, Ogre-ponderous arm
That hurleth Years unto their graves headlong:—
I grant thee all—accept—depart and feast.'

He ceased and sighed, still mourning for his son—
His long lost son six thousand years eloped.
Death saw not blood—Night only and Despair!
And Famine deep his every vital rent,
Whiles thus he roared harsh-gratingly to Night
As the infernal Echo's hoarse, rough blast
To Mockery's ear in cavern of the damned:

'I roved that world from fall of man till now,
Coursed her ten thousand thousand times around
Thro' storm, calm, heat and cold and life and death,—
Know well thy godlike son and where he reigns—
Ay, reign he will till Scythe of Death shall glow
All fire, and wake its hells of fury up
Fierce as last thunder of Omnipotence
And hurl to Ruin and Eternity.
Earth! idol of my soul I loved thee well!
Thou Earth! rich harvest field by Death-scythe reap'd!
I mark'd thy myrrh-perfumed vales and hills
With the dust-leveling besom of Decay,—
Creation-throned, Death made his proud seat thee,

And o'er great Nature reigned without compeer!
Behold Death driven from his high estate,
And Wo and Ruin hurl'd from mighty thrones!
God but unveiled his face smile-lit with Heaven—
Destruction's hosts were shadows 'neath His feet!
Retiring Hell howled out and fell Despair,
While Earth re-Edened leap'd to meet her God.
Ah! who 's omnipotent save Lord of Hosts?
Grim Death is but an agent of his will!
A servant in byways of Providence—
As Nothing's self in presence of great All!
I never felt so little until now—
Is the Devourer turning back to nought?
Annihilation come—Death would not be.'

He still'd and stood a blank—bewildered Wo
Without the light of Hope, or smile of Heaven—
Hell-grief communing with his wretchedness!
Despair, smote by the Worm that never dies!
Eternal Dial, thunder'd, and he woke
Fire-eyed, and roar'd with hatred and contempt:

'Death a day-labourer in the field of Time!

Mortality's slave serving for a crum!
Wast thou not mighty in the days of Eld?
Yea, who but God wrought wonders like to thee?
I was the thunder of the wrath of God
And ate Antideluvians at a meal!
Death rode the sword that o'er Jerusalem hung
With flame of vengeance and the frown of Heaven:
I marshal'd her sky-armies fierce and fell—
Fire-battles fought and rain'd their blood on man:
On Titus' sword thro' holy city swept
And smote the chosen Israel of God.
But now, alas! on Earth, Death is not known—
A gone-by tale unheard by mortal ear!
Not read of e'en in ancient chronicle—
Not named in all nomenclature of Time,
Nor shall, for a long thousand years to come:—
Millenial Day illumeth Earth as Heaven!
I saw it come bright as the smile of God;
Fair as Perfection's paradise of charms;
As Fancy's thoughts of Eden-loveliness;
Elysian fields of blessedness and peace—
Imagination's view of Deity!
I saw Jerusalem descend from Heaven—

God's Tabernacle dwelling with mankind,
And God with men, and they his children are:
Him, day and night they in his temple laud,
While pure heart's love of one vast people roll
To ear of Deity loud thundering on:
'The Lord Jehovah reigns, and kingdoms all
Of Eden-earth the kingdoms are of Christ—
Bride and the Bridegroom 's one, alleluia!'
Ten thousand hills reecho back the strain,
And hosts of Heaven loud answer in their strength:
'Eternal Sabbath of the Lord hath come!
Rejoice O, Earth! and clap thy hands, with thee
Salvation dwells and all thy tongues are praise!
Roll on thrice happy day of love roll on,
God fills the world as water the great deep,
And Eden smiles as Heaven—alleluia!'

'The world from blood and carnage God hath
cleans'd,—
The voice of Violence not heard on Earth
Nor is Destruction's mark on face of things:—
The whole world is the paradise of God,
The human race one brotherhood of men,—

No foe to harm, no spoiler to destroy,
For God hath victory over Sin and Hell,
And reigns supreme o'er Satan and his power.
I saw the Beast that fed himself and Death
On seas of Martyr's blood sink down to Hell
With weight of wo and wretchedness and crime—
All Inquisitions thundering at his heels!
Whiles dust of saints all glorified arose
In heavenly robes of Immortality,
To live and reign with Christ a thousand years.
And Sorrow, Sighing, Sin, Disease and Pain
Down to the Pit are hurl'd with dragons damn'd;—
Infirmity and Age and wretch'd Deformity
To Youthfulness and Innocence have turn'd
And sing and shout rejoicing in their God.
Grim War washed clean his hands from brother's
blood,
And man hath ceased to be a wolf to man.
Earth's heart doth hallow Virtue like a god;
Heaven's Peace is all in all; Religion bless'd—
That Vine of God from Eden's sacred bower
Now shades the world, and nought save Holiness
Is seen beneath its glorious canopy.

'Stately the Bride to meet the Bridegroom rose,—
How glor'ous are her steps—her strength the Lord!
Mortality is Immortality,
And Death hath nothing left him to devour:
Earth-heaven withholds from jaws of Death her
blood!
I've served thee since the dawn of time began,—
One favor asked—Eternity denies!
'Twas I that gave Oblivion kings and crowns
And monarchies and principalities;
'Twas I that gave thee all this sacred dust—
These wonders wondrous—all thou holdest dear:
Millenial Day shall I not then outlive,
And hear her ghost howl o'er Oblivion hills?
Say, who will give the Earth when I am gone
She fled? Canst thou leap o'er Eternal-wave
And give Oblivion to the light of Life?
Nay, this to thine own servant Death belongs,
Thy very humble servant—very true—
E'er true—obedient. Wilt thou reward?
I've faithful served six thousand years complete.'

He ceas'd and silence was that Chaos spake

All ear he hung him on Eternal-lip
And oned with answer yet in embryo,
Whiles moments in the orbs of centuries roll'd.
Eternity, stood like Nonentity,
Long buried in himself—Inanity!
Soul-travail in the mazes far remote
Heart-yearning o'er and mingling with his son—
His long-lost son, since Being's dawn eloped!
Grief was around him as Oblivion,
And wasteful Wo hung on him like a world.
Death's eyes flamed sulphur dens. A fearful light
His face illum'd that show'd him Horror's wreck,
Or fell Distraction grinning at the Shades.
Eternity, now rousing up himself
A moment woke as from a dream, and said:

'O! thou dread ruin of the wrath of God
Wilt thou not learn to fast? thou wilt—thou shalt!
For why should Feasting feast eternally?
Shall Gluttony of gorging make no end?
Intemperance swills not Bacchus' bowl for aye

And Drunkenness lays length of beastliness
With filthy hog in ditch, or mire, or slough
And starves to life and manhood once again.
Earth, days of famine well as plenty hath,
And man shall have long sleep for his short toil.
Hast thou not learnt to fast? sure infancy
Taught this. Thine own wretch'd mother gave
no food;
Thy jaws knew not to drain nutritious milk;
Long years elapsed e'er Abel's blood was thine;
Mankind had then one thousand years of life:
If tender youth for centuries abstained,
To what may not maturity attain?
Thou hast the blood of kingdoms now in store
And yet a-howl for cruelty and wo!
Thou goblin foul that claimest infernal birth!
Whom Hellhounds tore from horrid womb of Sin
And hurl'd forth—hideous! So huge, so foul
And monstrous, that Hell's sulphur-hearted king
Beelzebub fore'er unshaken—quak'd!
Hell-legions puzzled were to comprehend
And all the powers of Darkness shriek'd appall'd,
Till Indignation smote infernal doors

And Death curse-like rode Earth devouring Life
And stamp'd his mark of ruin on the world.'

He ceas'd, then spake and ceased to speak again,
While broken accents thundered like a storm
And Echo made Oblivion-mountains roar.
Then, stood one long, loud groan lamentable—
Soul-rending was his grief! A-howl for Time
In all the melting agony of Wo,—
Caves gloom'd around and Depth sighed out—
'Despair!'
Such doleful echoes smote the ear of Night
As made Eternal Darkness tremble, quake,—
Too vast for Homer's harp of fire to sing.
Grim Death, fell, fearful rose—Damnation in
His thoughts and Desperation on his brow:—
Awful as Ruin hurling thunderbolts,
And hideous as Hobgoblin all aglare
In sulphur den of Pandemonium,—
Red eyeballs glaring shot terrific fires!
Earth-leveling Scythe a horror manifold!
His right hand grasp'd the woful pest and woke
The beamy-vengeance flaming terrible:

But wasteful fury saw the dreadful mark
Divine, and paled like sun by moon eclipsed,
And look'd a beacon on Oblivion-hills!
With spirit-voice, convulsively it said:

'I can not—dare not smite Eternity:
Behold! Jehovah frowns and what am I?
Why threatens Death? Have I a traitor been?
What Fate herself could do have I not done
And faced the foe rejoicing evermore?
When I could smite have I not smitten dead
And gloried in the deed? Bear witness—Death!
Have I not served thee long and gallantly?
Thy Scythe O, Death! is faithful still and true:
With the great God at war shall I triumph—
From the Almighty-hand wrench Victory?
Let thou and I—the Grave and Hell be dumb,
For lo! we're conquer'd all and chain'd and
quell'd!
I'm not Death's Scythe by Sin and Satan forged,
But shepherd's crook that awes the stilly fold.'

It ceased to speak, and with pale Fear agleam

Low-crouching, hid, safe-nested in his beard,
Like fell Affright from coming of her foe.
Death, down to deep of all confusion sank—
A sea of grief and vast abyss of wo!
Supreme distraction and infernal wreck
Harsh growling: 'Must lay by, or—be laid by!'
His furnace-flaming eyes heart-anguish flash'd,
And thus he bellowed like an Erebus:

'Fate 's seal'd and all is lost! Death 's damn'd indeed!
Day of Almighty God 's e'en at the door!
O! who shall stand secure save God's Elect
In sunny robes of Immortality—
A-shout with joy on their eternal hills!
To old Iniquity and Death—wo—wo!
Destruction groans to Ruin in her cell,
And Vengeance is awake to war for aye
Damnation roars to Torment thunder-voiced:—
Hell is a Hell eternal in her wo!
Death asks not mercy—Hell hath none to give—
Ye fiends—I come! Ye damn'd—we meet, we meet!'

At wild uproar uprous'd Eternity,
Caught Death's last word while dying on the ear,
And interrupting, thus, in haste replied:
'*We meet!* 'Tis true indeed, and thou—a foe!
But wherefore? O! that I might prove a friend
And give thee back to carnage and to blood.'
'*A friend!*' Death thundered in his wild surprise,
'A friend—Eternity a friend! and how?'
He ceased, deep pondering. Interest most intense
And mute anxiety, jaws seal'd with seals.
Hot as Impatience-self bursting to hear,
Right forward bent to meet each word half way
That roll'd sonorous from Eternal tongue—
Pond'rous and mighty as an Earthquake's groan
Thus in Oblivion-shaking eloquence:

'Behold the vast, deep hollow of my side!
In fathomless abyss—chaotic wild!
Those mountain-heights of sacred Dust might house,
Or Earth, a revolution make complete,
Yea, planets, stars that world the heaven of space
Loose them therein as 'mid ethereal blue!
Behold me rent, torn, gone, and—fled away!

Myself no longer perfect and complete
As when Creation with Confusion dwelt.
In mighty void immeasurable as Night
TIME slept, and was,—that likeness of a God!
Filling all wondrous cavity within
Till call'd to king great Being's starry throne
And feed Existence with the breath of Life.
His presence gave to Pleasure's cupits joy,—
Charm'd into bliss Oblivion-quietude
Till groans! deep-wounded groans and deadly came
From one in labor sore and agony:—
I heard appall'd! nor knew what then had chanc'd;
No eye with fire celestial gleaming bright
Could pluck from Chaos-heart seal'd Mystery,—
Truths unreveal'd to Revelation give.

'Fell shrieks announc'd affliction deepning still!
Shriek answered back to shriek, and scream to
 scream
Lamentable and wild—wo-gnaw'd and damn'd
Till TIME knew—LIFE! His eye drank light of
 Heaven;
Blind Ignorance, fell from her throne abhorr'd,

And Wisdom sat upon his mind a god.
He heard the groan of Sorrow from afar:
His heart was melted to a fount of love,—
Soul oned itself with Wretchedness remote,
And spirit yearned to fly and be relief.
The wing of vast Impatience then he nerved,
While each succeeding groan new pinions gave.
Anxiety, in each wild look told haste,
And Agony sat on his brow convuls'd.
Lengths long a-down his lip hung piteous,
Whiles Pity's sighs met Misery's shrieks with tears
And gave to Mercy's brow the crown of God.
With Passion, long, his swelling silence fought
But fought in vain! Feeling's volcanic fires
Devourous flam'd within and would have scope,—
God-attribute! Mortals and immortals
Oppose alike in vain. The soul must speak:
A season it may be imprison'd, chain'd,
But last 'twill burst to sweep omnipotent!
Like some vast river stay'd by a strong wall
Till waters meet united in their might
And down to ruin hurl all 'posing things,—
Still on impetuous as Destruction leap

Drowning the vast-extended plain below!
So, councils deep of soul. The tongue must speak,
Voice thunder them, or Etna an eruption is.
They, o'er my son triumph'd and Hierarchs
Whiles God on Chaos breath'd the breath of lives.
Time spake, and fire on words of wisdom rode,
And eloquence, thus, like a torrent roar'd:

'Sire holy! Father dread—Eternity!
Long I have loved thee well, served and obeyed,
And I will ever love as I have loved
While firm foundations of Oblivion stand—
And may they stand for aye as adamant!
But—list! O! my loved father list! I would
Soothe Misery, wipe Sorrow's tear away,
Relieve Distress and chase the sigh of Grief;
Lull Care to rest, speak peace to Trouble's heart,
Bind up Affliction and Disease's wounds,
Heal Agony, hang smiles on lip of Wo,
Give back the heart of Wretchedness to Heaven
And plenty shower on Poverty and Want.
That groan again! O, how it rends my heart!
Soul-gnawing screams lamentable and wild—

Another! Yet another! long, loud, fell!
Thine only daughter calls with cries and tears—
Thy daughter CHAOS, eldest and first loved.
I am alone the hope of her despair,
The rose of health to her sore agony.
This, Prophecy of Eld, by thee oft conn'd
Thy constant wonder and delight, declares:
'*The great Jehovah—Heaven's eternal king!*
Shall on Old Chaos smile omnipotent
And make her pregnant. Let Eternal-heart
Now groan with growing life till Time shall fly
And pluck Creation from the womb of Nought.'
This Will Eternal travails nigh to birth,
And Prophecy loud groans to be fulfill'd.
Then haste me to thy child in her great need;
I pray to fly to Chaos' quick relief.
Their children's prayers kind parents love to grant;
Sweet Mercy's self is my own father's heart—
His daughter he will never cease to bless.
O! now to fixed decrees of Fate give heed,
Or Heaven's dread wrath shall blast us with a curse.'

'He ceas'd and seem'd Impatience wing'd for
flight:—
What could I when a daughter's woes besought?
What could I when my own loved son implor'd?
E'en prophecy was quoted! and it fell
From lips as thunder from right hand of God.
My son! my son! dearer than ought save God
I cried, we part as soul and body part,—
And I—content! Go—fly to Chaos—fly;
The number SIX, is set the sign thereof,
Break thou the seal and bid Creation be:—
But haste return, thy father's heart to cheer,
For I am Night and endlessly alone.

'Then nerved with an Immortal's might he rose,
Burst dark confines of his eternal home
And all asundered stood Eternity!
He heeded not, nor hearken'd to my groan
Tho' suffering more than Chaos ever knew!
But like some comet huge, high bounding on
O'er God-built orbs of Heaven and leaping Space
To light his fiery trail at every sun,
So Time rush'd a divinity in flight

To Chaos drear. Deliverance came with him!
And from that throe-belabor'd agony
The beauteous child CREATION, leap'd complete
Star-gleaming bright the glories of her God,—
The hand of God was pictur'd in her look!
Spring, Summer blossom'd on her face of charms,
And Eden gem'd her sunny breast with Heaven.
So perfect and complete the glory was
That Angels bless'd of God gave shout of joy
And Heaven's Eternal, seeing—good pronounc'd.

'But when seventh Morn had clumb the east all
smiles
The clasp was rent that tied maternal heart,
And from love's arms she leap'd—divine, entire,—
Embraced youth-smiling Time, and kiss'd and said:
'Thou of the rosey-cheek and zephyr-breath
And sunny looks bright blazing like a Heaven!
Thou nimble-leaping, orient-smiling Time,
O! leave thy father to his world of Night,
And I will Chaos my old mother leave
And haste to realms of glory and to light.
Parents so grum and homes so dark as theirs

Ill suit Youth, Beauty, Sport and Loveliness:—
Fair Beauty 's not admired, sweet Sport 's reprov'd—
Youth must be Age, or frown'd at and condemn'd!
To gain eternal pleasures is to fly—
Together fly—together live and love
And rule a kingdom of our own like God!
Behold, yon glory of the new-born Day,
Bright centre of revolving Planets eight—
Flooding all worlds with light of Deity!
Be that, the pure empyrean of our joys—
Our throne exalted where we reign supreme
Hard by the throne of the Eternal All
To lead the Star-hosts in their paths thro' heaven.'
She ceased, with look of love whereon hung soul;
Enraptured Time leap'd high for joy and said:
'Be ours for aye the music of the Spheres!
And glorious, too, and many be our days
As starry deities that dance 'round God.'

'He ended, breathing spring. Oned hearts and hands.
Like fatal arrows sent from Ogre's bow
Enormous and well bent, they outflew Thought,

And left Old Chaos and Eternity
Steeped in Distraction's tear and gall of Grief
To mourn their loss—deplore their flight in vain.
Avenge—avenge! O! right me of these wrongs,
These galling wrongs that deeply gore the soul—
O! bring them back fast bound in Ruin's chains
And I will be Death's feast in Famine's hour—
A peaceful rest from thy long labors all:—
Yea, I will lull thee quietly asleep
In Honor's Bed on Ruin's sacred Pile
Till God's Millennium of peace, joy, love
In arms of Night shall howl to Evil's Morn
Of Death and Hell and Devastation near!
Then Death, to vengeance shall awake again
And sweep from conquering unto conquest on—
Shake Earth, while I the golden harvest reap:—
One thousand years repose I'll grant thee Death.'

He ceased. Death bellow'd joyous agony:
'Hail, Chambers dark of Desolation, hail!
Black Horror! brooding Silence and Old Night—
All sacred wonders of Oblivion!
Thou Ruin's Pile of loneliness and peace

All hail—all hail! To me most welcome thou!
Death—ho! thou art divinely blest indeed—
In Honor's Bed I sleep to wake again
To wider horrors and to deeper woes!
The thought 's repast and gives to Famine food,
And vengeance whets sharp as the razor's edge.
Lo! Death shall forth again to shake the World,
A desert make of Eden-breathing Earth
And hurl Creation headlong down to hell.
Thy son I 'll bind in adamantine chains,—
Rub Life as cipher from the Book of Time:—
I swear to thee Time's self shall loose his name,
And plung'd to Ruin be—Eternity!'

Thus spake he loud, and would have spoken on,
But huge uprose Eternity—like God!
Full breathed upon the Life-devouring fiend:—
He sank. He fell as Andes huge, or vast
Olympus would if hurl'd aloft and dash'd
To Earth by Power Omnipotent. Dread lay—
One long unmeasured ruin in his length
O'er hill, o'er vale—sad Ruin's Pile the crown!
His desperate Dart slept cradled in his arms,

And his all-monstrous Scythe around him twin'd—
His only winding sheet, nor groan'd to fell
Destruction now, but seem'd like one in love!
And Earth knew Peace and Joy one thousand years.

BOOK V.

The Closing Scene.

BOOK V.

FROM Nothing's Chambers dire of Nameless Night,
Thro' all Annihilation's mighty void
Celestial-winged Vision sped as Thought—
Forth to the *Valley of the Shade of Death,*
Whose Mirror gave to view—THE CLOSING SCENE.

I saw Religion fall from her high tower,
And Virtue speed to her own native Heaven—
Thy spotless robe O, Innocence! defiled,
While Piety proclaim'd that all was lost.
Mourn O, ye Nations that adore the Lord!
Who daily walk with Him as friend with friend,
While shouting glory to the Lord of Hosts

Lament! weep! Vengeance' roar is heard afar,
Blackness of Darkness stirreth up herself
And Ruin's hosts come armed with many hells!
Ye woods! ye groves! ye everlasting hills
Resound—'Wo to inhabitants of Earth!'
Ye rocks! howl out, for Death and Hell are near.
Groan thou—O, Earth! O, wail with agony
For crown of Peace is falling from thy brow,
And Eden-glories flying from thy hills!
Thy cheek of loveliness begins to pale;
Thy joyous youth is wrinkling into age,—
Thou beauty basking in the smile of God!
Thy night is coming and thy grave is dug.
Great Nature! beauteous, God-made Nature—thou!
O! rend thy glories all—put sackcloth on
And down from thy heaven-home exalted come—
Prostrate in ashes rose-wreathed maiden—weep!
Pour out thy soul till Angels feel the wo,
For Loveliness decks but the tomb of Death.
Millennial Day is fleeing from the world—
Prophetic Sabbath, Jubilee of Earth
Three hundred sixty thousand years in length!
Lo! Angels are retiring on their clouds

And Christ and Martyrs home to Glory speed
And speak the reign of Horror nigh at hand.

The king of Day majestic walks the heavens
High-towering on superior and alone
With floods of glory blazing him around,
While waking worlds drink daylight from his beams!
Full-orbed immensity that crowns the skies,
Art thou the buckler of Omnipotence,
Or Heaven's all-orient eye down-looking—Day?
Art thou a smile upon the lip of God,
Or a reflection from the Heaven of Heavens?
Thou glowing witness of Jehovah's word,
How terrible the brightness of thy disk!
Thy God-created flame days Earth with light,—
What eye can gaze upon thee and yet live?
Heaven is thy pathway, light thereof thy rays—
Night flies afar and worlds exult 'round thee!
Art thou not a divinity O, Sun?
Of glories brightest and the most like God—
From thy face floodeth glory as from God's!
High o'er Starland thou walkest like to Him—
Art thou its light? its life? its—Almighty!

In thy broad blaze great Nature lives for aye,
And Darkness' self is vivid light 'fore thee!
Behold, thy presence is Eternal Day,
Thy absence—Night and Chaos come again!
Thy awful presence speaks a Deity:
Thou sweepest in thy strength omnipotent
A dazzling splendor burning on alone—
All-brightness from whose smile Daylight is born,
Whiles pale and lost sink all the hosts of heaven!
Thou flame of Day and glow of stars by night—
World-life and deity of Universe
Had I not heard of God I 'd worship—thee!
Pilgrim of Heaven! art journeying to God?
Wilt thou grow old as doth Mortality,
And call aloud in thy great need, on Death
To lull thy wearied feebleness to rest,
Or, is thy race from Being's birth to aye?

Thou must run down thou mighty clock of Time—
Grow dim with death thou lighter-up of worlds!
Yes, Day-eyed Sun! thy glories shall be quench'd
For God will breathe upon thy face of fire
And thou shalt out as taper in a blast.

Thou prodigal of light! e'en now thou sit'st
On Old Hesperus' brow like Glory's crown
On forehead of Archangel, luminous,
Calling thy far-extended beams to rest
That mantle clouds in purple and in gold.
Weary thou sit'st! there 's sorrow on thy cheek—
Sink, sink to night and bid the world farewell.

Earth smiles an Eden, lovely wooing sight;
Her fairy-bowers laugh out—Elysium!
Where Romance wild in solitude arrayed
And Spirit-shade and balmy Coolness walk
With rose-cheek'd Health in rural quietude,
While music-footed Zephyr breathes of Heaven
And loads his odor-wing with Paradise
Love-romping with the Flowrets of the Spring
With fire of inspiration in his song.
In their own fatness, wide her broad Farms spread
And promise give of plenty to the world;
Life-feeding Fields toss golden heads aloft,
And ripening harvests wave—wealth to mankind;
Elysian Gardens all laugh out to flowers
That load the bee with sweets the air with balm;

Soft, shady Lawns inviting to repose
Where Loveliness flower-crown'd with Beauty romps,
And Children cherub-cheek'd gambol in love,
Or lilies-like lay—careless flung on grass.
Her little, round, proud Hills do people plains
Where the swing-making Vine snake-like climbs
trees,
And grape-hung boughs bend—purple luxuries!
Broad Rivers, silver-veining flood the scene—
On rumbling roll and talk to shelly-shores
Where shepherd's pipe gives music to the groves
Whose leafy-lips kiss zephyrs passing by.
High, light-reflecting Cliffs, where sunbeams glow
With Glory's fires like Angel-bands above;
Huge well-like Vallies, sombre in their depths
Where dewdrops sleep the live long day away.
Dark Glens in all their native wildness lone,
Where Muses and Apollo rove at will
And give their souls to Poetry and Love;
Elf-haunted Caves of Terror and of Fear
Where glow-worm's lamp is ghosts to cheek of
Gloom,
And Spirit-shadow, grum, midnights the noon

While Spectre Blackness holds her festivals.
Grim Dens! where Morn with Darkness wrestles hot
Whiles on his throne eternal and alone
Affrighted Night grows faint and sick least Heaven's
Seraphic Light (the smile of Deity)
Should welcome to his home the god of Day,
And give his bed of Sleep to Care and Toil.
Earth's blue-robed Mountains are the Landscape's
smile!
They hang afar dream-like, and spirits seem
Of Fairy Land deep-shrouded in grey Mist:
Their rock-crown'd heights heave high their heads
of snow
Above the storm-cloud's desolating howl
To live forever in serene of Calm
And bask in smile of Peace, sunshine and heaven.

Embosomed lonely in the woodland skirts,
Ambrosial Pools paint all the breeze-moved trees
And sleep with heaven upon their sunny face;
Live landscapes speak from their bright mirror'd
look—
Clouds fleecy play on bosom pure of pearl!

The silver-footed Streams walk grassy lawns
And to their silvan shores talk lovingly,
And snake-like Brooklets, glide, quiet along
While pebbles dance to sweetest harmony.
Gay, skipping Rills a-jump dance o'er the stones
As things of life, and joyous as the Hours!
Creeks, leap from rocks and change to Waterfalls,
And Whirlpools dimple o'er the River's cheek
Whose waters roar to rocky depths and roll
A clear, cold length of majesty along
Whiles laughing waves come rippling to the shores.
The crystal-bosom'd, rivers-drinking Lake
Is Nature's mirror bright reflecting heaven!
It breathes dew-drops to flowery vales afar,
And vapors gray rise curling from its breast
All dotted o'er with fleetly flying ships
That softly kiss Old Neptune's briny face
And joyous play upon the glassy flood:—
They seem like spirits of a fairy world
Melting apace to nothingness and air!
Vast Ocean dim in misty distance floats
The king of Waters, monarch of the Floods—
Live Romance all unveiled to eye of Earth!

Creation thou of God watering the world,
Thy living, fishy-waves are many poems
And their world-music roars eternal on :—
Those lovely Isles are children at thy breast !

Great Nature wears full Eden on her cheek,
And all her flowers are rosy smiles of Spring.
Vast Woody-wilds deep auburn'd o'er with Shade
Where fawns are feeding in their innocence,
And marriage-loving Vines are wed to Groves
In loved embrace close-clinging to their joys,
While fruit nectarean clusters all around
In rich profusion—feasting to behold.
Huge Forests give their branches to the cloud,
And wave storm-wrestling heads in dizzy hights—
Beauty in boughs and music in their leaf.
Like arrows, Pine and Fir trees dart aloft
Spear-heads that pierce the sky—half way up
    Heaven !
Each bough is curtain'd round with wavy-leaves
By Wisdom's hand and perfect Beauty made
When most they sought their matchless skill to
    try.

The vale-embowering Elms like heroes war
With Summer's sultry fires that parch the heath;
And spread shades wooing in their blessedness.
The kingly Oaks in majesty up rise
Rock-rooted and cloud-capt, crowning the plain
With house-like trunks and woody heads of storm:—
A grand old Oak years-grey and bald at top,
Cloud-high throws woods-grown boughs heavens-
reaching up
And stands sublime the sentinel of hights
And mighty herald of Antiquity.
The water-loving Sycamore, white, smooth
And branchy, freckles o'er the river's face
And clings to stony shore grotesque and wild.
The Laurel-groves unfading branches give
To breeze, and weave their own immortal arms
In Glory's wreaths to crown the Poet's brow.
Doth not yon graceful-waving Willow talk
Of gesture perfect unto Eloquence,
Whose action times with Zephyr's heavenly song?
The Aspen with perpetual-motion leaves
To Melancholy lisps in mystic notes
And with the passing spirits—dialogues.

The jolly-tripping, spirit-footed Air
Feeds with the breath of life the joyous Hours
And gives the World-harp heavenly rhapsodies!
Young Zephyrs romp within love-wooing bowers
And tune to harmony the sweet bird's throat;
They curl at will the aged Ocean's beard—
They chase the flying billows o'er the spray,
And lift on high the fragrant head of flowers:—
Those fairy-footed Winds have each a voice,
And melting as Love's sigh dissolving hearts;
Soft-breathing children, they, of Tempest are,
And spirit-like play—tiptoe with the Hours.

Birds speck the scene and give the Landscape—
voice!
Their laughing souls are innocently glad:
They sing their sonnets from the breezy-groves
To love-mates wed to their rich wealth of eggs,
Or on wings glitter brilliant gems of air,
And like the all-hued rainbow—paint the heavens!
The merry Lark rings ditties to the spring
Till skies speak out like a rich peal of bells,
And air all music fills the dome of Heaven.

The jolly Thrush in canopy of leaves
Wakes up wild-warbling woods to rhapsodies,
And Catbird with love-stories weds a mate.
Bees, music-wing'd buzz to their fields of toil—
Kiss lip of Flowers to find the honey's home,
While Butterflies flit—wing'd Poesy of air!
The white plum'd Pigeon streaks the skies with light,
Full-blooming lotus blossoming thro' heaven,—
Down drops on Earth as snow-flake from a cloud!
The Parrot talks to Echo and the rocks
In language not his own, and understands
His greek like learn'd professor at the schools!
Moss-woven nests of symmetry and skill,
Defying Art and human workmanship
Do gem the woody-hills all chirpingly!
The cooing Dove pours out full soul to God
In hymns of thankfulness for breath of life,
And numbers o'er in tear-steep'd elegy
Each mournful day the Savior lay entomb'd,—
She singeth thrice and Sorrow's heart is rent,
She stays her lyre to give her soul to grief.
The Humming-birds o'er flowers of beauty rest
While nectar-sipping bills are drinking life,

Then sightless buzzing as bullets—shoot air!
In branchy hawthorn hedge dance twittering Jays,
And eyes and hearts win of their lady-loves
Whose dulcet notes charm Echo into song.
Woodpeckers with their blood-red helmets on
Smite hammer-like their heads upon a tree,
And hills have voice loud as the bugle's roar;
Woodcocks with mallet-head and trumpet-beak
Awake afar the forest-thunders up,
And make aloud the tall, dry beach resound.
That nimble Squirrel sits erect as man
With umbrella-tail high o'er his head,
And rasps his nut high on his dizzy limb:—
Now, lightning-footed leaps from bough to bough
Eyeing the hawk and barking at the storm.
The towering Eagle sails in Ether's home
Floating like Fay in island of the Bless'd,—
Still upward—on! to make Cloud-land his own:—
Now at bo-peep aplay with man in Moon
While sunbeams romp gold-sandal'd on his wing!

Health walks o'er all the Eden-breathing Earth
And heaps up roses on the lap of Life;

On Nature's face the smile of God is seen,
And cheek of sweet-lip'd Flowers the blush of spring :—
Sweet *Flow'rs!* the smiles, joys, blisses of young Dawn
That jewel Nature o'er with Eden Loves
And man's path on to glory and to God!
They are all balmy with Elysium,
And they paint Earth with colors dip'd in Heaven.
The Lily turns from Zephyr's kiss of life,
And veils in dew her Sylph-like loveliness:
Fair Virtue's emblem—child of Modesty—
Perfection pure as ringlets of the Morn!
Thy face is likeness of the Seraphim,—
In Beauty's robe array'd and Love's own smile!
Thou Eden-joy and white-robed Purity—
Thou Angel of the Vale, there 's room in—Heaven!

The giant *Mountains* rise—sweeping the sky!
The world's loud boast, her fadeless glory, pride
With romance clothed and all alive to fame!
'Gainst base rock-rooted, warring surges leap,
And angry billows dash themselves to foam.

Forests of fir are bending from their breasts,
And rocks moss'd o'er with age show their white
locks
Dim-twinkling down thro' vapor and grey mist.
Their gulf-o'erhanging cliffs look fear and dread,
Where Rivers change their names to Cataracts
And leap with earthquake-shock and thunder-roar
To the celestial fields their spear-peaks rise
Sublimely lost in chambers of the snow,
And bird of Jove rests there his wing of heaven.
Play ye with sunbeams at the fount of Light?
Do ye behold young Morn's awaking smile?
Saw ye the king of Day asleep on couch?
The majesty and awe of Earth's greatness—
Sublimely-speaking-grandeur-thrones of gods!
God-monuments amock at old Decay!
Antiquity that time the more divines!
The Tempest stays his storm-car on your breast,
And Whirlwind raves round ye an idle breeze:—
Ye laugh the awful Hurricane to scorn,
And heaven in fury is a thing of nought!
Your Earth-broad shoulders cleave the battle-cloud,
And thunderbolts fall harmless as a rain.

Like Deity ye tower—sweeping alone
Whiles Vengeance hurls to ruin all beside;—
Ye frown upon the Lightning's fiery hell,
And stand unmoved while God is passing by!

Now, god of Light upon his golden car
The dimeyed Day to yawning gulf of dark
Oblivion rolls! and sable-vestured *Eve*
In all the sombre deep of Mourning robed,
In her heaven-state of pomp and power appears,
The funeral of expiring king to grace
And give his ghost to the Eternal Hills.
Death-bed of dying Day is all asmile
Like a meek Christian going to his God:
How many-voiced the lovely Landscape sings!
Play-loving leaves dance prattling to the breeze.
The Insect-swarms float on the placid air
Their little wings all music as they hum!
The honey-laden Bees buzz home to hives;
Crickets begin to serenade their loves.
Sheep-feeding Shepherds pipe heart-melting lays;
Loud-bleating flocks ring Hunger's supper-bells.
Echo, aloud speaks Cuckoo's name to rocks;

Bob White talks love to Miss Quailina's ear
To paradise himself in her pure heart.
Eve-hymning Larks song-breathing and choir-voic'd,
On quivering pinions float celestial heights
And pour out heavenly sweetness of their hearts
Till Ether's soul melts with the melody:—
Those airy warblers seem like Angel-harps
Divinely tuned to psalm the Savior's love!
The rocks peal unto rocks, hills answer hills,
Groves talk to groves and woods ring loud to
  woods,—
Reechoing heaven resounds with harmony!

Young *Twilight*, now veils Beauty's cheeks with
  pearl,
And light with shadow blends soft as love-hearts,
While Supper gives soft-curling Smoke to dance
On cottage chimney-tops like Ghosts of night
And walk the skies light-footed as a Dream.
To slumber's downy couch sluggards retire.
Sweet Zephyr gives his lip to cheek of Flowers
And romps with Lily like a child at play.
Shade-spectres walk the moon-lit dells like Fays,

And star-tears hang—jewelling the cowslip's ear.
Bright, fleecy Clouds gem the cerulean plains
And float—the slumb'ring Seraphim of Air!
Winds fan with half-closed wing the joyous Hours
While rustling groves breathe melody and love:—
Health is the air and harmony the breeze
Music in bowers and moonlight on the hills!

How bland the starry-smile of *Evening* is!
Mother divine of Silence and Repose,
Thou dost remind me of bless'd Spirit-land
Where all is calm, serenity and peace!
Heaven hangs with ornaments her pure concave;
Awide her mantle spreads spangled with stars—
Heaven's world-embroider'd curtain all divine
That hides from mortal sight the Heaven of Heav-
ens,—
Sun-starr'd as Eden with all beauty was!
The *Sky!* in its blue-length of glory spread—
Expanded wing of dread Immensity
And flight sublime of vast Infinity!
The God-extended magnitude of heaven—
The might of God and right hand visible

Deep crown'd with moons and ponderous rolling
Worlds!
Stars! there ye blaze heaven-glories sparkling
bright
Thick sown by hand of God o'er field of Space,—
The twinkling stars night-born and fair as light!
Are ye the gems of God's eternal throne?
Eyes of Creation lit at Glory's fount?
Heaven's laughing daughters dancing o'er the sky?
Spirits aglow with immortality?
The happy Bless'd a-leap with joy 'round God?
The silvery gleaming Seraphim of Eve,
Or daylight-fac'd young deities of Night?
Angels a-wing thro' Ether's wide domain
To glorify infinitude of space?
Heav'n-thron'd ye reign God's sentinels divine—
Divinities that preach—'A God beyond.'
Twinkling ye visit worlds with smile of Heaven—
Immortal Purities by no spot stain'd!
God-'llumin'd lights where Day-eternal lives
Flooding out glory like a Deity!
Suns lit with glory burningly alone—
Celestial suns! where orient heavens revolve

With song harmonious as Zephyr breathes
To ear of Angels, or of Cherubim.
Fix'd *centres* bright by worlds encircled far,—
Yea, worlds on worlds in paths remote from these
Find worlds on worlds gem their fixt-centres round,
And spheres on spheres in crystal fields of light
View spheres on spheres in loftier stations still
And mightier globes 'round mightier Day-stars burn,—
Systems on systems orbit vaster orbs,
And greater lights flame out to greater fires
That shine to planets circling other suns,
Whiles planets, still, 'round higher heavens revolve,
Till mounting Space they crown the infinite
And they have found their one great centre—God!

The poet of the grove—sweet PHILOMEL!
Within rose-bowers deep-nested and alone
Thou makest Eve more lovely with thy love;
Thy strains come forth by rose's breath perfumed—
The soul's own music and the spirit's voice!
Thy notes are tun'd by Inspiration's self
To all the melting melody of song.

Till Echo mocks the star-eyed night away.
Thou spirit-stirring Minstrel of the wood,
Pour out the inspiration of thy soul
To make Eve lovely and thyself beloved
With voice that speaks of Eden come again!
Pour—Pour! Bright Spirits answer near and far:—
But—stay! Eve's ear is wed to harmony!
The vales rejoice—the hills speak out and live,—
Silence is charm'd and utters forth a voice:
'Thou wast renown'd in Eden's sacred bower
For song divine and poetry and love—
And Angel, still, the music of thy lyre.'

Eve steeps her eyelids in the dews of NIGHT,
And drinks the roses from the cheek of Day.
Night's veil hangs o'er the landscape's living green,
And sable mantle shrouds a hemisphere!
Her eye distils the pearly tears of Dawn,
And jewels o'er the princely breast of flowers.
Tir'd shepherds sleep sweet-dreaming of their God,
And birds are wed to leavy-rests till morn.
Visions air-wing'd adorn the hall of Dreams;
Shadow and dusky Gloom stalk thick as ghosts.

The dog loud howls to spirits passing by.
The fire-flies scatter starlight thro' the vale,
And artificial day wakes up around;
The merry glow-worm with his lamp new trimm'd,
Now promenades his own true-hearted mate
And lights the rose on cheek of his espous'd.
The breezes tune wind-harps to ear of Night.
The skies come down on mirror'd fountain's face,
And bays, lakes, straits and rivers all laugh out
To see their bosoms' glow so n uch like heaven's.
The fleecy cloudlets float balloons of air
O'er ocean-skies all flooded thick with suns
Gleaming the glory of the Heavenly world.
Star-armied Night 's a-march o'er fields of blue
High towering on majestic and divine:—
Star-fields! ye spread out blue immensity!
These are the heavens God made, and no star dimn'd!
Those lit-up orbs innumerable to man.
Clad in their robes of fire the meteors flame,
And shoot like spirits to Eternity:
A comet trails red length of light along;
There lays wide-splendor of the Milkyway,
And lo—the Moon! stay, I will sing thee, love!

How sweet the borrowed smile of Luna is!
Her eyelight's glow is Darkness' banishment—
Noons Darkness into light more loved than Day!
There 's spirit-light in her celestial smiles,—
Sweet drop of glory on the brow of Heaven!
The full, round eye of Night with glory fill'd,—
Thou Ark of Light! loved sister of the sun
And star-crown'd daughter fair of Paradise,
Thy downy softness glorifies the skies,
Thy halo-flooding cheek reflects Day's smile
And flowings of thy silver locks light heaven!
Thou art world-loved high Empress of the night,
Earth's fairy-robe and Evening's blessedness—
The King of Day is pictur'd on thy face!
Thou show'st thy virgin loveliness full orb'd,
And walkest in thy brightness—maid of Heaven!
Love-crown'd and smiling as God's own Redeem'd,
And Night is Eden'd with thy joyous beams.
Thou pure and lone sweet dweller of the sky—
The beauteous handmaid of the glorious Sun
And Angel-laughing lady of the heavens,
I hail thee Queen of Starland evermore!
The Planets leap rejoicing in thy smile,

Their pearly eyes gleam joy looking at thee:
Lead on Heaven's virgins in their airy walk
To play with Ocean and to woo the Tides.

Sleep—dull-eyed god! with death-like sceptre spread
From sea to sea reigns monarch o'er the globe,—
Life 's cradled on his breast! Repose is Earth,
And Silence dwells on lip of Solitude.
Grim MIDNIGHT frowns at dread Eternity!
A change is felt in Being's mighty soul.
Time's clock strikes twelve, and Nature roars out—
'DEATH!'
Bells from their brazen lungs wring forth dead
sounds,—
One din of bells, dogs, cocks and raven croaks
The ghostly ear of Night with bedlam fills,
And robber Owlet's hoot hath demon in 't!
Volcanoes smoke and flame fire-mouth'd as Hell.
Mist, Vapor in their Jack-a-lantern robes,
With Gloom and Fog saw air with misty deaths
Begriming Ether's crystal fields of light.
Pale stars seem lost—wild-wand'ring o'er the skies!
High, lone and cold the white Moon floats along—

Stands still in heaven,—falls back, and climbs again
Blood-orb'd! Sweet Philomel wed to her own
Wild, Echo-wooing rock caws like a crow,
And mock-mouth'd Echo is a grave-yard's knell.
Cloud-mountains roll their ebon cars on, up,
That foul Night's cheek and blot affrighted skies,
While Darkness blackens round cimmerian.
Old Ocean wrinkles at the wild Wind's howl;
The willow's length of limb lashes the blast;
Fork'd Lightning flaps, and shows fire-wings of
wrath
In sulphur-rumbling bowels of the cloud,
And dreadful Thunder hardens there his bolts
For deadly blow at brow of Guilt and Crime.
Bright, star-eyed faces beam 'twixt wing of clouds
That hide from Earth retiring Mercy's smile
Where Angels sigh and Seraphs weep for Man:
Like many fires, pale Ghosts light up grave-yards,
And flaming Cherubs glide thro' Night—mete'rous!
Amourn are Spirit-groups upon mid air,
Whiles heavenly-voices to Earth's poles proclaim:
'The world's Millennial Sabbath hath expir'd;
Satan, a little season is unloos'd,—

Speeds to deceive four quarters of the Earth,
To lead forth Gog and Magog with their hosts
In number more than sands that shore the sea
To dreadful battle—ARMAGEDDON call'd :—
A crisis big with vengeance is at hand.'

That sound afar is Death's deep dismal groan !
Behold, he wakes ! awakes with all his woes—
From arms of Sleep Eternal leaps and howls !
His eyes white-rolling flash as lightning's glare,
Their sheeted flame athwart Eternal Night's
Dark den speeds witheringly, and lo—she quakes !
Hell howls ! and wider ope than Ghosts have known
Flies gates of adamant ; and fiercer, damn'd
Than Satan's ear e'er heard, awakening Wo
And Vengeance growl for prey, while Death roars—
'Blood !'
Yell-famin'd and gaunt Hunger 'yond a grave !
Abaddon is let loose to ravage Earth :
Destruction's host is armed with many deaths
Loaded with bolts horrific, Ruin stands !
Roars Devastation like a storm for prey,
Whiles Desolation with his Hadean-breath

Beneath his load of indignation bends—
Swings his Creation-uncreating-club!
Towards mankind their woful coming is,
Impatient now to smite with demon ire
The angel-brow of seraph-smiling Life,—
To turn all loveliness to loathsomeness,
And Beauty give to winding-sheets and worms.

'Round Death, thoughts famin'd swarm tumultuous
As scowling fiends, each roaring for its prey:—
Darkens in wrath and speeds—World-ruin on
In Terrors clad and horror'd with his Woes
A sea of deaths—a vast abyss of hell!
He flies to Earth—Heaven-guarded bower of Bliss!
Where blooms divin'd the rosy flowret Life
Immortal Seraph ripening for the skies!
As forest-bending Tempest is his flight—
A Desolation making desolate!
He sweeps Hell-armied on dragon wings
To wage a demon-war with works of God,—
To ruin kingdoms and to blast the world
And pluck Creation from the smile of Heaven:—

Storm, Whirlwind, Midnight, spectre all his path,
And Earthquake Terrors his tomb-opening way.

And when his foot of bone press'd rock-ribb'd Earth,
Back shrank she trembling from the loathed kiss
And heedless of her beaten track cours'd heaven.
Great Nature stood aghast and shook and sighed;
From hill and vale came forth deep shrieks of
Life—
Ethereal concave echoed to the groan.
As Earthquake shocking nations was his stride,
Ghosts shriek'd and yells of Damn'd came forth
from far—
The tomb was heard to utter forth a voice!
Black-banner'd Wrath spread out on air. Fate
lower'd.
Affrighted planets stared and stars eclipsed:
Creation's bosom throb'd. Life-pulse of vast
Existence flutter'd to be gone—was still!
Great Being's soul was a death-agony.

Grim Death, saw, heard, and howl infernal gave,
And breath'd Simoon and Pestilence and Plague.

He stood high towering o'er a steeple's hight
Mid fearful terrors of a thunder cloud—
Eternity dim-dawning thro' his form,
Daring to war with thunderbolts of God!
His Scythe immense flam'd in his right hand's grasp
As lightning God's, to drain deep sea of life
From Nature's heart, and smite Creation vast
On God-exalted throne and hurl headlong
To deep Oblivion and Eternal Night.
His lean, lank jaws by wasteful Hunger gnawed,
Half ope and watering all impatient stood
To close on man and feast on human gore,—
His goblin-face as grim gaunt Famine grinn'd!
His comet-eyes aglow roll'd deadly-dull
Their baneful fires and ghosted Eden-air—
Portentious heralds of fell Ruin near!
He, sombre, deadly stood agloom with Hell
As Condemnation shrouding spirits damn'd
In fell Death-shadows of Unrighteousness.
Earth darkened with him! Rocks and caves wept
tears:
His frowns gave midnight's cheek a deeper die.
A lion's thoughts while leaping on the fold

Were his,—ay, sharpened daggers newly whet
Red-gleaming vengeance and athirst for blood.
His heart was havock and his spirit fire;
His soul all tempest lightning-wing'd with wrath;
His jaw's crash thunder; terrible his roar—
In his loud howl was heard the fate of Earth!
A rattling roar around about him went,
And where he breathed was pestilence and death.
Air curdled at his touch. Mortality
Was poison'd with the sight. Earth quak'd at
tread,
And Palsy's smite fell on the face of things.

Like tempest lashing spirit of the deep,
Death's frantic gestures were, which spake aloud
To near and far distracted eloquence,
While thunder-toned he thus soliloquised:

'In Heaven's arms lock'd and sweetly sleeping—
Earth!
Sleep on—to wake up in eternity.
Satan is loose and Hell unbars her gates,
And Death 's awake to give thee sleep indeed!

Ay, sleep thy fill e'er Vengeance howls thy knell.
How heavenly rests this bright Millennial-world!
An Eden in Prosperity's love-smile
That basks with Joy and Happiness and Peace
At Plenty's wide-spread board of luxury
Sipping pure bliss from Pleasure's fount and
Heaven;—
Weep—weep—there is a cloud upon thy brow!
Thy bliss shall broken be,—but in its stead
With liberal hand I give large recompense,—
Death, Hell and Wo! Choose thou to bargain thus?
Grim Death will have it so—let that suffice.
For each joy-drop, I give a sea of tears.
Fly—Peace! and angel vestur'd Joy be dumb!
Thou rapture-winged Bliss! away to Heaven
Thy native home to visit here no more,—
Thou Happiness! hence to Oblivion
And leave mankind to chains of Fate and Wo,
For cloven footed Sin, Iniquity,
Black Crime and dragon Wretchedness and Pain
With fell Disease and Pestilence and Death
Fiend-claw'd and fang'd come desolating hells
To ratsbane Life and make the Earth one grave.

Earth-joys! how soon ye wither at my touch!
Earth-pleasures! feeble as is Frailty,
Where are ye when I breathe? Dust of a tomb.
Lo! what a field is opening on my view!
Great Being rich—to harvest-fulness ripe,
All, all stand ready for the Scythe of Death!
Death reigns Life-monarch on forever-more
God-like and wasting as the Elements!
Gaunt Famine gnaws, but Plenty's smile I see—
Eternal feasting near Death starves no more!
Unbounded fields of loved Mortality
Do proudly wave their golden heads on high
And promise vast profusion crowning all;
But Death's time-killing frosts what shall escape?
Ho! I will plunge me in the mighty maze—
Reap Fallen Nature's harvest as a field
And feast on Life with gusto of a king.
A world of princes schooled by heavenly hosts
And fed on manna for a thousand years
Invite King Terrors to right royal feast—
Magnificent repast—the marrow, life—
Carnage of Worlds! He will not fail to come:

'Tis light to eyes and music to my ears—
Death prides to think of such a luxury!

'Blood—blood! Ah—*blood!* that name so long unheard
Sounds strangely sweet to my awakening ear
And fills the leaping soul brimful of bliss;
How more melodious than the song that sings
'*Heaven dwells with Eden-Earth a thousand years,*'
Tho' by Archangel's golden harp announc'd!
Thou sweetest cream of richest luxury—
A luxury beyond all luxury,
To my gaunt jaw a chosen spicery!
Ichor of soul and honey drop of Life,
O! how I thirst for thee—delicious *Blood!*
Far richer to my taste than nectar-milk
That woman's breast for infancy distils.
My sluggard Scythe awakes at thought of thee—
Brightens to reap the flowery fields of Life,
To crop the roses from the cheek of Time
And pompous-strutting god Mortality
To hurl from Fallen Nature's heart headlong
To kindred dust and dire Oblivion.

'The vast world sleeps—near pit of her despair!
Red vapors shroud the land as flames of Hell;
Grim clouds rain blood, and havocking the night
Damn'd Spirits rave in thunder-roaring cars
To smite Millennial bliss from Nature's heart
And riot with her glories and devour.
O'er hills and vales a dismal murmur runs;
The caves loud bellow and huge mountains groan,
While Echo bedlams caverns with her yell.
Wo, Fate and Destiny on dragon wings
Fly Earth around with Doomsday in their frowns,
Whiles Life's great Angel speeds—shrieking despair,
And fiery Spectres ghost the gloom profound.
With sharpen'd fangs and talons whet on Hell
Uproarous Demons rend the dull sick air
And cloud-like hang on brow of night—black'ning!
Hope flies from man and leaves to Earth—Despair.
Bright Seraphs talk of death to all below,
And weep, and vanish as they groan—to God.
The world is Satan's seat, Apolyon's home—
A sister-neighbor wedded unto Hell!
O'er fallen Earth reigns Death a god supreme,
And he shall crush her with his weight of wo.

'Morn's sentinel sweet Venus wakes dim eyed;
Feeble her ray as lamp that lacketh oil,
And heaven's bright loves all sicken in the sky.
Daydawn brings Woes that slumber not nor rest—
Life's thousand years of glory then expires!
The ghostly Past, as shadowy as Vapor's breath,
At breathing Present looks Oblivion,
And rings her death-bells at Futurity.
Earth's day is short—her very name is wo,—
Awake O, Earth! Death whets his Scythe for thee,
And Hell 's agroan for souls and I for blood:—
Blood—blood! acquaintance with thee I 'll renew—
Lo! Death begins his works and mighty toils!
Toils—toils! my pleasure, food and pastime, ye,
Supreme delight, joy, bliss on evermore—
Life-goring labors, ye shall have no end!
To deeds horrific rise my daring soul
And fit examples high of heroism
To Spirits damn'd and fierce infernals give,—
Haste, smite the world and like grave-yards devour:
I 'll make wide deserts thro' the heart of Life
And spread Sahara out from sea to sea
Where Simoon sweeps hell-flaming with my rage.

'Fiends, Imps, Hell-hounds of Wo—safe bottled up!
Wrath-vials! Ye I pour on sea and land.
Disease, Affliction and Distress and Want
Toil, Care with Cruelty's death-lash in hand
To scourge Man o'er broad road of Wretchedness
Till tomb receives and Hell holds fast her own.
Here, Vial is of Desolation fierce
Loud groaning as the regions of Despair
To earth bright Genius, to Oblivion Earth:—
Hah! there growls Vengeance and Eternal Wrath!
Ho—Terrors! like to ye, poor man ne'er dream'd,
Earth knows not of—Affliction's back ne'er felt!
I set ye free—depart, begone—fly hence
Ye Imps, for Luxury's table fills the land,—
Away—Death follows hot in the pursuit.'

He ceas'd, unstopp'd Wrath Vials ruinous:
Forthwith out pour'd Woe's countless multitudes
That darken'd air and hid the vaulted heavens.
Black Evil, as a vast imbodiment
Of Night, spread sable wings that blotted skies,
And o'er the world hung brooding like a pall;
Dire armies of Disease flew mail-clad,

And thick as swarms of bees from Summer's hive.
Fell Tribulation, Anguish and Remorse,
And demon-steeped Calamities of Hell
With their fire-pains and groans and sighs and tears,
Storm'd forth Sin-legions fierce of utter wrath
Whose breaths were poisons breath'd from fetid lungs.
In zenith altitude they pause—darkling!
View'd unobservant Earth from pole to pole,
And whet their sulphur jaws, tusks, fangs and claws
On burning Rage and flaming Fury's ire,
Till wing Infernal like a whirlwind swept
To his own work, each separate and apart,
Howling as ravy Damn'd by Scorpions
Pursued with whip of pestilential fire.
They seem'd one moving cloud immense and dread—
Awaking eye of morning was eclipsed!
More numerous they by far than locusts were
That famine gave to Egypt's grassy plain.
The sound of mighty hosts were many storms
In lightnings clad and arm'd with thunderbolts:
Death's ear awoke with woful melody,
And grinning like a cavern, he exclaim'd:

'Ho! Devil-music feasting to Death's soul!
My Demon-warriors! in your turn rejoice,
Rich, fat feasts after our long-famine come!
Break now your fast on ruin of a world.
Take thou thy fill of blood O, Cruelty!
Till Vengeance' self shall cry—'It is enough.'
Thou tempest-breathing Indignation! grind
Mortality's clay-tenement to dust:—
Destruction—on! like mighty Flood of old
Impetuous in thy course till groaning Earth
Lies strangling in the slaughter of her sons.
Dread Cholera—hence! and tempest Nature's heart,—
In death-cramp dismal grasp the Universe,
Oblivion Life, and Earth a death-bed make.
Hell-tooth'd Affliction! riot in Time's path
And give to Being's soul last-agonies,
Till deep-mouth'd Wailing shall forever wail!
Knee-knocking and bone-rattling Ague, fly;
Hence, big with utter wrath, loath'd Palsy, hence,
And Devastation! shake Creation's nerves
Till tottering jade shall tumble to the tomb.
Fiend-hearted War! mark Kingdoms for thy crown,

And call the imps of Inhumanity
To set thy cloven foot on neck of man—
Haste, brake thy age-long fast on human gore.
Ye raving Winds—awake! Ye Tempests up—
Up from your cavern'd beds with all your rage
And in your fearful strength arise and fly—
Rend, rend the stubborn hills—lay forests waste
And mountain seas and oceans make one wreck!
Fell Earthquake—mighty prototype of Hell!
O! swallow islands, continents in wrath—
Gorge Nations at a meal and groan for more
To glut your vengeance and your fury quell
Till heart of vast Existence rends piece-meal
And Desolation is made desolate.

'O! be affrighted Earth! my wrath is fire—
The fire of indignation that burns worlds!
Lo! Eden-charms fall withering from your brow—
To ruin like a whirlwind thou art hurl'd!
Fierce Plagues fell-struggling at my girdle hang
And only hell shall e'er be found of thee.
Thou pale, lone Empress of the Night—wail, weep!
Thy light-reflecting face shall turn to blood,

And thy maids mourn around thy couch of death.
Ye stars! that peal out wondrous harmony
To paradise the great Eternal's throne,
Be mindful of your ways—watch well your dance,
From paths stray not, for I can reach ye too
And headlong hurl to Chaos back again
As Bacchus' Lethean cup, inebriate.
Creation! howl aloud, Destruction 's near
With Vengeance' bolts red-gleaming in his hand,
And door Eternal stands a-jar for thee.
Quake thou O, Time! Son of Eternity,
I 've adamantine chains and bolts for thee
That groan e'en now to bind thee hand and foot,
As I, to give thee deep Oblivion.
All Hell—arouse! wake horrors of your fires,
And back on rusty hinges, brazen gates
Fly quaking, rattling, crashing, thundering,
And let Apolyon forth armed with thy hosts
For lo! it is the Dragon's time to reign!
Yawn wide O, Grave! Life's roses to receive:—
Victorious Death! on, woo and wed lov'd Earth
Tho' Bride of God may sicken at the sight!
The lonely widow's moan, the virgin's shriek

And infant's cry be music to thy ear:
The stormy screams and groans and sighs and tears
Of pity-melting Agony shall speak
Sin's reign supreme and Death's Millennial feast.
I 'll drain from Life-heart its deep sea of blood—
A Wo-confounded world with hell-rage ride
A tempest-breathing pestilence red hot
To make Time hurricane—all Earth a tomb
And bask in Nature's ocean-misery.
Behold O, Earth! the King of Terror comes
With all his Woes and Horrors, Terrors-crown'd—
His course spreads Desolation down to Hell!

'*The sign—the sign!* Behold the sign O, Time!
Thou World! behold thy own death-warrant seal'd.
Roses of light, wide scattering o'er the bright
Pavilions of the East, aloud proclaim
The stately steppings of gold-footed Morn,
At whose love-smile Millennium shall end.
A rising sun, Death's day of vengeance brings—
Haste, rise O, sun! and glorify the world,—
Arise, but not to see God's Son on Earth—
Death's jaws instead and grinning to devour!

A Scythe that playeth like Archangel's wing,
Athirst to bathe in purple flood of life
And ocean Earth with the Death-luxury!
I burn, the hateful footprints to erase
Made by gold-sandal'd Sabbath of the world.
Where Heaven's great King, the Lord of Glory
tower'd
In day that Eden's loveliness excelled,
And led the Angel-vestured Martyrs forth
With Virtue's white-robed chosen sparkling Heaven
One thousand bright, God-numbered years complete,
I, Death, will walk with all my Hadean woes
And hell the Eden as I did of old
Till not a gleam be found on this side—God!
I 'll light mine eyes with livid soul of fire
That Sleep inglorious with his hateful mask
Or curtain black of magic mystery
Eclipse them now no more, nor yield again
To Slumber's lap of loathsome quietness
That hell-crown'd king and giant-greatness—Death!

'Lo! Love and Mercy's banners are roll'd up,
While Hell's black flag of Vengeance is unfurled

And with the lashing gale wars smitingly!
I see—Death-sign! wide-painting earth and heav-
en—
One long blood-day of feasting lights the sky,
As bless'd to me as Paradise to man.
Millennial harvest now is ripe to full;
Grim Death shall reap the crop and fill the tomb:
It grows Starvation's claws more deadly, fell,
Whets Famine's fang and sharpens its dread point;
My every vital gnaws to gnaw the world—
I fly to mark Creation with a blight.
Hell! ope thy jaws, grin horrible and wild,
I 've a God-world to feast thy famin'd mow!
O'er Earth I sweep, and every step digs graves—
I crush a thousand lives at every stride!
Ho! Death hath nought to fear forever-more!
My demon Woes have circled Earth around—
I 'm growing now almost Omnipotent!
Earth! whither flee when Death is every where?
My new-dug-grave-jaws ope world-wide for food
And Life shall drink in death at every breath!
Behold! I now will crush the universe
And hand to hand war with Infinity!'

He ceas'd. Aside with Hell conversing stood;—
He stood in statued-dignity supreme
Dumb, stiff and cold as a stone monument,
And with his horrors gloom'd the atmosphere.
One horrid load of wild intentions now
Roll'd thro' his mighty bosom like a sea,
And frightful fiend seem'd ocean at full tide—
A growing ruin swell'd to bursting nigh!
His cave-like jaws terrifications grinn'd;
Air, into poison 'round about him turn'd,
And Life beheld and sadden'd at the sight.
Thick Darkness veil'd tear-showering face of
Heaven,
While Night, deep-shrouded in dark clouds of Gloom
Lay down his wretched corpse at rosy gates
Of Dawn, and groan'd aloud and wept and died.
Peace, saw, and saw no more! Hope fled, and bless'd
Religion sped to God day-flaming like a sun.
Loud roar'd Death—Etna in eruption he!
As meeting thunderstones his fell jaws crash'd;
His eyes, fire-splendors of the burning noon:
Rock-rendingly as storm swept howlingly—
Hell by his side Destruction at his heels!

BOOK VI.

The Closing Scene.

BOOK VI.

THE wearied stars are lost in fields of blue;
The cold, pale Moon looks down wan-fac'd despair;
Dawn melts away at mournings of the dove,
And Day dim-gleaming lights up all the heavens.
Snow-drops have couch'd them 'mid the leafy-grass,
And thro' their veils of dew, like stars—twinkle!
The rising sun of half his glory shorn,
Sickens at sight of Heaven-forsaken Earth,
And eying Death with look of wan despair
Seems the All-seeing Eye in tears immers'd:—
He wraps him in his robe of deity
And floods of glory flame ineffable,

Whiles waking Nature's smile like summer glows
And worlds afar are gladdened with the god!
Earth, sparkles in her dewy loveliness,
While God-robed Light trips spirit-footed on
Awide o'er her soft lawns as bright as flowers,
And all her groves sing praises as it comes.

The sun pours noon on sisterhood of worlds,
Then stands appall'd in heaven—falls back! flames, dimns!
He pales and quakes as frail Disease death-couch'd—
Throws robe of high divinity aside
And from the face of Day looks—a blind eye,—
On heedless rolls regardless of his course.
A deadly Mist veils hoary mountain-brows;
Afar grey-coated Fog curtains the sky,
Where sunbeams wander pale as Feebleness
To gaze on Nature's dying loveliness
With sickly look of green-eyed Melancholy.
To poisonous Vapor pestilential fens
Give birth, and troubled waves of marshes, ponds
Send fever-breeding Damps sick'ning the land.
Diseases, walk awide smoke-breathing Swamps,

And seem like many deaths upon the wing:
An Ignisfatuus dim and distant romps
And purple winged flies buzz o'er the plain,
Whiles dark-fac'd Shadow wrapt in weeds of wo
Stands by his cave somniferous and dark
All dragon-mouth'd and gaping like a hell!
Fearful ghost-Gloom on stalks grum, mournfully
Up ravines dismal and obscure and wild
That shroud eyelids of Day in pall of Night,
Whereon curs'd Demons grin deformity,
And Fiends obscenely dance to gaunt wolf's howl,
Owl's hoot, the vulture's shriek and wild-cat's squall.
Hell-dragons fierce hum dismal out on air,
And fiery Spectres glare on wings of wind.
Hyena's fresh-dug den gives Terror's crown
To hill-side's craggy steep where tangling wilds
Glow with the madden'd tiger's glaring eyes.
Voracious leopards growl surly and mad;
The panthers cry, and grim, gaunt wolves howl
blood,—
Affrighted Bruin scrambles up an oak!
Half hid in clefts of rocks fire-serpents hiss
The fetid venom from their baneful mouths,

And on their cloven tongues hang poisons—green!
With bite-like features of fell terror, dread,
The Rattlesnake lies coil'd to smite down foes,
And Blacksnake glides a creeping-darkness on
Death-poison dropping from his forked tongue,—
The Rabbit's safety is his flying foot!
The dreaded Porcupine stands all aloof
With his ten thousand spears of death erect;
The hedgehog deeply digs a safe retreat
'Twixt two huge rocks that brow a precipice.
The robber Hawk is swifting thro' 'mid air
With squalling blackbird fluttering in his claws,
While clouds of birds do tempest him about
Proclaiming vengeance to the murderer,
And throw themselves as bullets at his head.
The evil brooding Raven sombre, shy,
To mate caws out his lessons vile of blood.
The Owl hoots fiend-like in dark-hollow home.
Sky-cleaving Condors float cloud-like thro' heaven
And scream as furies, then—down-drop on prey.
Frog-armies, long, loud, wild and hoarsely croak
To their aquatic graves shaking the marsh.
The Brook lisps mournfully to Sorrow's heart;

Niagara's earthquake-waters roar afar.
Uproarous Seas talk with Eternity:
Whales with their island-backs spot the huge Main,
Then, tempest ocean with their goings-on.
Clouds ride on giant Winds presaging Storm,
Beglooming Ether's heavenly home sublime,—
Up thunder-wheel'd they roll blotting the skies
And mingling with the hoary Ocean's beard,—
Sky-leaping waters blossom into foam!
Thunder is heard low-bellowing afar;
Chain-lightning telegraphs the storm's approach:
Mad, grim the scolding Blast bounds o'er the heath
And combs the forest's lofty head in rage.
Fierce-rending Gales wake all their trumpet-harps,
And voice of dismal Vengeance peals aloud
Chastising Nature with the curse of God:
Fierce Whirlwinds scold Creation while they live
And howl themselves to Chaos back again.

The mighty *Spirit of the Storm* is fledged!
Comes howling on aloft and fury-wing'd—
Arush to mark an awe-struck World with death.
Birds tuneless cling to lashing haw-thorn hedge;

Beasts howl and rush from smiting wilderness.
With warrior Winds fight Forests gallantly;
Their giant arms aloft fall crushingly.
The shiver'd woodlands show their storm-split heads.
Deep-rooted firs, the pride and glory, growth
Of centuries, leave their brothers in the wood—
Mount up aloft thick-peopling all the cloud,
And like fell Ruin wing'd, speed dreadful on
Till Desolation's wreck marks Earth's extreme.
The fire-eyed lion with his mane erect,
Mocks the loud roaring thunders as they rend
Proud oaks that bow not down to angry Heaven
While God in terrors clad is passing by.
The mad Sea down to depth, with fury boils;
Her giant heroes rise Olympus high
Rending her rock-bound home and battling Heaven!
Lost ships, her mountain-rolling billows crown,
Their top-masts tilting with man in the moon
Till down they plunge to everlasting night.
The anger-lifted Ocean's mane stands up
Erect in rage—lashing aloft! Rough face
Wide frowns, and dismal her roar rides the blast.
Upon her boisterous billows Ruin leaps—

Destruction in her mighty surges rolls.
Fire-flaming lightnings ride on desperate wrath
Of groaning Heaven, with red-arm'd thunderbolts
Fierce hovering round the frown of brows—bellowing!
The sombre raven wings mid-air and drinks
The zigzag terrors as they flash along,
And croaking loud sees death in every bolt.
The Tempest's arm falls with a desert-blight;
Huge mountains quake and the rent rocks have voice:
Heaven is one flame of indignation fierce,
Whiles Storm-fiends breathe in frenzied violence.

Earth quakes to find herself in Satan's power;
She shrieks aloud to feel hell-fangs at heart,
And stands—wild-wondering where her Lord hath flown.
Man wakes surpris'd to know the novelty
Of pain and agony; sighs, weeps to hear
The maddened Tempest's desolating howl.
The people mourn instead of praising God;
Fear, trouble, lamentation come in place

Of joy and bliss and songs of thankfulness;
Gaul fills the cup where milk and honey flow'd,—
Grief's arrow barb'd is fluttering in the heart,
And fountain-eyed weeps Mourning o'er the world.

Once, Adam walk'd with God in Eden-bliss;
Rebellion grew upon the tree of ill;
He ate—death to the world and fall of Man!
So, second Eden falls like first—headlong
From God's love-smile to very gates of Hell,
And brings the times of peril on all flesh.
The Nations to seducing Spirits lend
A willing ear—doctrine of Devils learn
Till alienated from the life of God
They shun Religion and renounce their faith,—
Despising those more holy than themselves!
They choose not now the ways of Righteousness;
The path of Holiness is not delight;
The creature more than the Creator serve—
Vain-minded worshipers of sinful selves!
Love Sin and Pleasure more than they love God—
Quite given over to Lasciviousness
To work the works of Sin with greediness—

By vile Affection wedded unto Hell.
God-haters they,—inventors of iniquities,
The worshipers of idols, silver, gold
And wood and brass that see not, hear, nor walk—
In league with Old Iniquity and Wo!
Their consciences as with hot iron sear'd
And understandings darkened into night
Speak:—'Spirit-eyes put out—blindness of heart,—
The heart-corrupt resisters of the Truth
Denying power of Godliness with oaths!'
They strive to banish thought of God from mind,
And fill soul full of all unrighteousness:
Their minds and consciences defil'd as filth—
Abominable to God, and—reprobate.

Behold! heaven reddens with the wrath of God!
Now, turns to frowns and seven-fold night as soon,
Then, Summer into Winter quick as thought,—
Creation feels the change throughout her works.
Cold Boreas comes ice-wreath'd on frozen wings,
And swallows chatter to the chilly air;
Snow-storms howl winter-anthems chillingly
Through full-leafed forests wailing mournfully.

Grim Horror rides the wasting Elements;
Wo comes to try his might and horrify;
Hell wakes in fury and impatient quite
For universal desolation seems.
With sea-wave wrinkles Vengeance plumes his brow
Where earthquake-frowns storm—turning men to
ghosts!
Grim Death rides many-shap'd devourous all;
And hand in hand with Dragon takes his way
With grave-yards strewing Earth at every stride!
He measures now his woful way along
By his own greediness, and spreads one wail
Of ruin, wo and every hideousness
As forth he sweeps with hell-howl on devouring.
Earth, bids farewell to heavenly Blessedness,
Weds her with fell Iniquity and Wo
Whiles Satan grins and numbers her his own.

How is man fallen from his high estate!
The beautiful to Sin and Hell gone down!
Poor Man that lived in Eden-bliss and reign'd
A thousand years with Christ, invulnerable,
Is now estranged from God and hope of Heaven!

Disease and death hang on him like a curse;
Sin, Wretchedness encamp around about;
Calamities and Wo bend him tombward,
And many deaths he dies in dying one.
His days but few, and full of troubles are;
He, shadow of a shadow seems, whose life
Depends upon existence of a breath:
His every wish—voice of a dying sigh,
And every joy—reflection of a tear!

God made Man upright, in him spirit breath'd,—
Unto His servant never gave a want
That Earth was not found able to supply.
Contentment fill'd his heart with peace, joy, love;
With thankfulness he gave pure soul to Heaven
And fed each wish with manna from on high,
While Happiness benign walk'd hand in hand
With Wisdom and fair Virtue up to God.
But Man in sable council sat, and plann'd
Rebellion foul against the Holy One
That made Creation and pronounc'd it good:
Inventions many sought he out to make
The world a hell, and labor'd hard and long

Devising death to Immortality!
Then peacock-strutting Pride with head of wind
Came forth and stood auxiliary to his aid
Mortality's tormentor to become,
When, Life's few wants to Legion multiplied
Till Earth was found too barren to supply!
And Vanity! O, hide thy head—Hellhound!
(The advocate of all licentiousness
And royalty's apology for vice)
Came to undo, and make man wretch'd for aye;—
To recreate the works divine of God,
And the death-stab to Peace Eternal give,—
Yea, make Mankind as Sin and Death and Hell
And base Desire, would have them made—*devil.*
Thus, sable council sat and long devis'd,
When fell Deliberation and Debate
A new creation gave of monstrous birth:
Into a world of wickedness and sin
Now turn'd that Satan-seat—HEART OF MAN!

The code of laws made by the Prince of Peace,
Which rul'd by love and purified the heart
Abolish'd is by Satan, Sin and Man.

Philosophy, Morality and Right
And Liberty and Peace feel deep the stab,
And Nature's groan is heard to world's extent.
Religion is by law prohibited,—
Man hates Religion and forsakes his God
By tyrant Passion led and appetite.
Blind Prejudice smites Reason from his tow'r,
While Falsehood plucks the tongue from mouth
of Truth
And slanders neighbors with his lying words.
Hypocrisy puts on her mask of night,
Oils up anew her cloven tongue of lies
And wins a ready way to heart of fools,
Whiles Confidence and Candor have no place.
Justice is cast to hungry lions in their den,
And Faction, Villany and Wrong walk Earth
Awide corrupting all of human-kind.
Integrity is broken on the wheel;
From judgment seat Equality is hurl'd,
And Arrogance high-seated in his stead.
Love, Mercy, Equity are all dethron'd
And Hate and Vengeance triumph at their fall.
Pride, Crime in purple and fine-linen strut,

While Honesty is scoff'd at and despised.
Illustrious Worth bows down to Fortune's sway,
While Lewdness sits in state and talks with peers
Far-fallen and low-minded as himself.
Ambition, Folly, Desperation, Hate
Speed desperadoes howling to destroy,
And climb to Honor's seat and rule domains
And sceptres grasp of universal power.
Kings are made slaves and Emperors servants,
And servants kings and bondmen emperors,—
Lords, gov'rnors, stirrups hold for former slaves,
And Princes, bows on back of Foppery tie,
Then paint the cheek and black the shoes of Pride—
Receive for pay loud curses and sore stripes!
Bless'd Freedom 's chain'd to banish'd Liberty,
And Bondage beats his bondslaves on to death.
Oppression's power falls wasting all mankind;
His iron rod on drives his servile droves
Thro' bedlam-life of slavery to the tomb,
And bless'd Humanity is in her grave.
Fell Tyrany enthroned reigns absolute,
While Murder sceptres his right hand of death;

Power's nod, the signal is for massacre,
And Earth's great heart wide pours at every vein.

The good are met and banish'd all to lands
Afar, and housed with Echo in her rock.
The jails and dungeons are illustrious made
By crowded throngs of princely prisoners.
Health, Happiness, Prosperity are chas'd
By sore Affliction, Misery and Misrule;
And Pestilence, assuming different forms
Gives death and ruin to the Elements,
Whiles Wretchedness and Sorrow fill the land.
Economy and Temperance leave their homes,
And Prodigality and Beastliness
With nameless crime wild-riot thro' their halls
By day and night devouring and devour'd.
The wicked profligate and libertine
Conceal'd in skirts of Night's eyeblinding cloak,
Dark Midnight's constant conflagration are:—
God's holy temples fall by lawless mobs,
And Virtue by base Immorality.

On every heart is thron'd blind Ignorance,

And many temples rude do steeple skies
Sacred to her, tho' call'd by Wisdom's name!
Intelligence is hiss'd at and despis'd,
And Nescience wide roves from sea to sea.
The light of Mind by Folly's darkness veil'd,
Flames out no day to heaven the world, and bid
Sage Wisdom from chaotic sleep awake;
But Error blind and base Stupidity
And fiend-indwelling Wickedness owl-eyed
With God-forsaken Bigotry on roll
Their one cimmerian night o'er all mankind
Till midday sun of Knowledge is eclips'd,
And God-bless'd Piety with look of Heaven
And full salvation in her sunny smile
Is bosom'd with her God, and Anarchy's
Loud howl of hell is heard to Earth's extreme.

Man strives to lose himself and his own soul,
The visitations of high Heaven forget,—
Yea, those who dwelt with Christ the Lord on Earth—
With Savior walk'd one thousand years complete
Cry out—'*There is no God, or Heaven, or Hell,*

And no Millennial Day hath ever dawn'd!'
And those who prove the falsehoods to be false,
The demon Infidelity rends sore:—
When a devout and holy man is found
Fit subject he is deem'd to crucify!
Fidelity is down to dungeons cast,
Or fetter'd stands by base Deceit condemn'd
Till Torture takes the martyr to his stake.
Truth, Wisdom, Piety are hunted down—
Fall like autumnal leaves and trod to dust
Beneath the foot of Mobs and lawless Power:—
All sacred things are trampled in the dust,
And hideous Vice, Profaneness, Blasphemy
Arise on dragon-wings aloft, and course
The guilty Earth with impudence of Hell,
While Man's loud plaudits rise and smite the skies,
And high above—climb holy hill of God!

Hail, holy word! world-sun and Wisdom's noon—
Wisdom above all wisdom of the world,
Celestial radiance beaming upon Earth
At whose bright blaze soul-darkness is no more!
The spirit's lamp in prison-house of clay—

God-light wherein the nations sun themselves!
The map of Heaven and road to Zion's hill!
Instructor wise that schools us for the skies,
Whose heavenly manna is the life of man—
Man's guide to Immortality and God!
The staff of strength in hand of Frailty
Mortality's wild-wandering foot to guide—
All hail, thou—HOLY BIBLE of the Lord!
Thou hast illumed Earth long, gloriously,
And taught the saints to scale the mount of God—
Led Virtue in life's narrow path to Heaven,
Tak'n Humbleness from dust to great reward,
Giv'n Hope to smile o'er gibbets and the stake—
Bless'd Faith to eyelay God thro' Sorrow's storm
And bidden sinners flee the wrath to come;
But near accomplished now thy work below,
Thou hast grown old—fast fading from the world,
But not by Infidelity destroyed!
End-seeing Prophecy groans to be full;
Soon, thou shalt crown the Judgment Seat of God,
And the *Lamb's Book of Life* wide opened be
And all things judge according to their works:—
Thou sittest now upon the night of Time

To light Creation to her wreck and grave,
Then, try her ghost at the Eternal bar.

The Holy Bible bless'd forever more!
Hated by Sin in every age and clime
While one fool 's found to do his father's will.
Aloud the people roar against the Light,
Of—'contradictions' talk, absurdities
And romance wild and fable monstrous!'
Condemn to flames and burn it when they meet
Tho' much they fable love! They, story seek
And novelty the world around, and spend
Their lives and fortunes all to seize the prize:
When find a story of enormous growth
That bends their evil passions like a bow
To highest pitch, and makes them quite forget
Their own immortal souls and Heaven and Hell,
O'er it by day and night they pour entranc'd
Feasting on wind—rejoicing with great glee!

An enemy to self was never yet
A friend to God, nor can have hope of Heaven.
The Bible shows to man his ruined state—

Far-fallen and corrupt, sin-blacken'd heart,
And bids him fly to saving blood of Christ
And wash Pollution's every stain away:—
He flies to burn the Book—the word of Life!
The great physician of his soul destroy
That freely offers everlasting health!
This sacred mirror shows to man his heart:
He loathes the glass because that heart is black,
And seeks to break for showing his true state!
Hates sacred Light, not Sin who is his night,—
So would a devil! Men by willful crime
Make Word Divine their fearful enemy,
And therefore are they deadly foes to it,
With hate of Hell they scoff the sacred Truth
Because it is not what they wish—a lie!
Ay, prophesy it will not—good of them,
But evil ever—Wrath forever-more!
To see a Bible, now, in brother's hand
Signed warrant is of death. They crucify
The readers of the book, to kill the book!
Ah, fools! that Bible thunder-voic'd declares
They are but fighting with the Lord who said:
"The Heavens and Earth shall pass, but not one jot

Or tittle of my Word, till all 's fulfill'd."
How then can imp, or infidel destroy?
My soul's one book! Hand-writing of my God!
God's Will to men by Inspiration giv'n
Declaring them the heirs and sons of God!
God's Bible—painted speech that speaks to eyes—
The body visible of His pure thoughts
Revealing—Light, Life, Immortality
And full Salvation to the sons of men!
Thro' wrecks of Time and Ages thou hast stood
And no jot dimm'd by years, man, fiend, Earth,
Hell—
Nor can, till Heaven itself shall be no more.

Prince of the Power of Air in terror reigns
Exalted high above the name of God,
And Death and Villainy in hearts of men.
Fell Sin down looks on Earth with gorgon eyes,
She banes her widening path to death and hell
And gains applause and universal fame
That wins her ready way to soul of kings,
While Vice and Immorality hell-born
And Satan-bound hot-follow her in rear,

And hand in hand with swine-like Filthiness
On speed the praise, loud boast and wonder wild
Of all, excelling far—Brutality:—
Hot chase of fool'ry! Folly is the cry!
Mankind pursue her both by day and night,—
Man strives with man each other to surpass,
Till all in turn by Folly are pursued—
Down hunted and devour'd eternally.

The ties of country, kindred, love are sever'd,
And Friendship's chain is broken utterly.
Contentment, Joy and Happiness and Bliss
Live only in rememberance and dreams,
And Righteousness, Worth, Honor, Honesty
Are nursery-tales and fables of the past.
Trust hath no being, Confidence no place;
Business stands still, Society is not
And heathen Barbarism deem'd politic.
Unpeopled cities to waste places turn;
Where tower'd a village grows the wilderness,—
Towns, deserts and ghost-haunted Ruin's home!
The pauper's cry and clank of maniac's chain
Instead of vesper-hymns fill all the land:—

The stake now stands where stood the church of God;
Jails, gibbets rise where bless'd Benevolence
With Love and tender Mercy dwelt enshrined
And pour'd out heavenly blessings on mankind
That worshiped God with purity of heart.
Blank Poverty gaps famine-mouthed on Earth,
And Famine grins grave-jaw'd at human kind:—
Their hovels, dens of wretchedness and want;
Their wisdom, spirit-blinded ignorance,—
Gangs brutalized, wild—savage-wandering!
The shriek of Violence is daily heard;
Adulteries, rape, untimely births frequent.
Man seeks by day and night the life of man,
And those that Murder spares are giv'n to hand
Of Cruelty to torture at her will,
And mercy the severest vengeance is:
Revenge and Fury den them in the soul,
Base Degradation hangs upon their brow
Bending mankind to earth—digging their graves!
The human heart to desperation turns,—
Transform'd to demon, Man defies high Heaven;
Iniquity and Crime with harlot's face
As lions rove with gory Vengeance on,

And Wickedness reigns o'er the world as Hell,—
An all-pollution—Sodom and Gomorrah!

The genial Seasons change, and Year's return
Is broken utterly. Day's eye looks blood.
Eternal Wrath and Indignation fierce
Make glow the heavens as flaming furnace hot
And roar to Man of Doomsday nigh at hand.
Grim Night like an infernal Dragon huge
Down rusheth from the frown of Heaven cloud-wing'd
While Darkness palls the Universe at noon
And howls—Earth wed to Wretchedness and Wo.
Uprousing in his rage dread Earthquake wakes,
Opes dismal gaping jaws and yawns and groans
At his last gasp—all-ruinous as Death!
Impetuous flies in desolating car—
Graves kingdoms in his wrath at every stride
And crushes towns and cities in his ire;
The mountains totter and the caverns yawn,
While wide world trembles, rocks from pole to pole.
Clouds burst, and Thunder leaps athwart foul air;
Red Lightning in her seven-times heated forge

Death-arrows hardens and bolts ruinous—
Preparing all her fierce infernal stores
For crush of Nature and the death of Worlds.

Grim *War* is fledged, and marks his gory way
To lands remote, and piles the mountain-slain.
The sword forsakes its sheath, and resteth not;
Battle the world and Pestilence the breeze,
And every coming moment breathes—despair.
Nations in bloody conflict, nations meet;
Kingdoms 'gainst kingdoms rise and fight and fall—
One people is another's death and grave:
But hottest flames mad Battle's wasteful fires
At EDIONA—City of Refuge!
Where Freedom wooes sweet Peace by night and day,
And all the banished dwell with Liberty,
And keep the Law and read the Holy Word,—
God's chosen, set apart to do His will
And be his Witness in the world below.

Virtue's beloved and the espoused of Truth
Clad in the saving robes of Righteousness—

Condemn'd and banish'd for their zeal and faith,
Came to ZIONA'S ISLE of pearl and gold
And safety found from Wretchedness and Hell.
They met each other with a holy kiss;
They lived as brothers and their friendship grew—
Heart wed to heart entire, their love—woman's!
Religion was their guide and God their friend—
The narrow-way lay lovely to their sight
And fed their souls on joys of the Redeemed.
God's bless'd! And they grew mighty in the isle
And loved Ziona was their little Zoar.
Vast forests fell. Fields ripened in the sun.
Wide-spreading farms chased woody-wilds afar
And laughing Plenty blossom'd like a bower—
Down shook her blessings raining on the land,
While Thankfulness as incense rose to Heaven,
And Peace and Joy on tiptoe clapt their hands.
God's temples clumb spring-glittering up the
skies;
Towns jewel'd o'er the vallies and the hills,
And cities were—thou EDIONA—thou!
Remote from Evil and a world of wo—
From Wickedness retired to be with God,

Where Virtue hath her shrine, bless'd Peace her
home,
And Freedom's banner floateth o'er the free.
Mid vine-clad hills spring-fed and grove-embower'd
Fair Ediona towers Bride of the Prince—
The virgin daughter of the God of Heaven!
Where Justice smiles to Mercy while he rules;
Where Arts and Science give soul-wing to mind;
Where Learning counteth stars, Wisdom flies
heaven,
And Genius strives for rivalship with gods.
Ziona, faithful, 'mong the faithless stands
Proclaiming God and Resurrection Morn,
And feast on joys that take fast hold on Heaven:—
She stands secure amid the Pestilence
As Goshen stood encompass'd by Ten Plagues.

But earth's full eye of evil on her roll'd
Redning with sulphur flashing of fell hate
Till envy turn'd the human heart to fiend,
Then Nations swore to Nations in their wrath
To be her ruin—her devouring fire,
And give her ashes to four winds of heaven.

Mad Slaughter rose with murderous arms aloft,
And Persecution, Vengeance, Massacre
Breath'd Battle-spirit from their sodden lungs
To gore World-heart and be her wreck and grave.
In boats and crafts with all the woes of war,
Five hundred thousand dreadful warriors came
And burst upon her gates with wild uproar;
But Ediona—Heaven's true hero stood
Invulnerable to Envy's storm and Hell.
Religion was her strength and God her tower;
Her soul was peace and purity and love—
The Lord of Hosts her trust and sure defence
'Gainst man and powers of Darkness all combin'd.
Three circling years the Nations fought complete
Loud thundering at her gates by night and day:
Stern Heroism strode desperate forth, but fell,
And Bravery, Bravery met and was undone—
The mighty, nerveless lay pil'd, bleeding 'round.
At post stood Duty firm, and hand to hand
With Valor fought but found his grave e'er night.
Power nerved his might and swept forth like a
storm,
But saw a foe superior and died.

Strength met an arm that level'd him with dust,
And Greatness found a greater and his tomb.
Art, Toil beneath their task down sank, expir'd,
And Genius search'd her stores and found but
dreams,—
The might of Stratagem was idle wind,
And Wisdom, falling, groan'd wise plans to death.
All fatal arts of war were tried in vain,—
The Nations did but—fight, flee, fall and die,
Whiles holy city stood—God's Ediona still.

Upon Ziona's wall Grim Death appears!
His direful form of famine looks disease
And battle forth with pestilence and wo,
Whiles Dissolution gurgles from his throat.
Destruction-arm'd and Terror-clad he stands
A statued Horror—Fate is in his look!
His eye the fiery lightning's sheeted flame,
And arm the lowering thunder's desperate might.
His laboring brain a carnage-house of wo
Haunted and fed by fury of his soul,—
Death-dooms are seen wide-written in his face!
Diseases thicken 'round about him grim;

Plague, Pestilence in fatal shadow stand,
And 'hind him Desolation and Despair
Spread their domain thro' Chaos down to Hell.
A sight so fell that Darkness midnights 'round,
Ghosts shriek, and Echo bellows out—GRIM
'DEATH!'
The weeping moon thro' mist looks blood, and wrath
Of God on cloud and sky flames sulphurous,
While thus to self he growls as Spirits damned
To mountains, rocks that hide them from the Lamb:

'Grim Death yoked with the Whirlwind to destroy!
Lo! we have cours'd the world nine times around,
And cry of all my Imps is still—'Havock!'
Hell, Death and Sin have tainted all below—
All but Ziona! saved by Him whose arm
Is terror, and whose name 's Omnipotence.
When will her thousand years of life away?
Earth's holy Sabbath hath departed long,
Yet God preserves his Ediona still!
Ah! why reserve this city to Himself
While Ruin sweeps all quarters of the world?
Is Tyrant partial to these hills and plains?

These founts of song and streams of melody—
Brooks pouring through the heart of Solitude
And mirror-lakes that paint as Spirits—Heaven?
Those Eden-groves where beauty weds the eye,
And golden fields whose harvests feast the sight?
High mounds where Seraphs bathe in founts of dew;
Ghost-wilds of Darkness waving midnight-locks,
And caves whose night on slumbers evermore?
All these are odorous with millennial bliss,
But are they bright as was the sunny south
When God's own presence bless'd the mundane
Earth?
Christ dwells not here as in the days of peace,
Nor Angels one them with the sons of men;
But will He yield entire this jewel'd-love?
He will:—Death 's written upon all save soul,—
Content thee Death—all conquest is thine own,—
Grim Death shall king Mortality for aye;
I bring the Plagues of Egypt to thee, jade!

'Almighty, now hath hidden Him in clouds!
Then clang of arms is music feasting soul:
War is the joy of my heroic heart—

Mad war out bellows many devils damn'd!
Earth-wasting War! howl out for havock—howl!
To vengeance sweep—drown thy hellfire in blood
Where Fate meets Death to slay a million fools.
Chase soul from man thou world-devouring War!
Death mounts thy murder-car—red Battle-fiend!
We 'll desert Earth and make this globe a tomb
From conquer unto conquest is our stride
And victory and vengeance all our own.

'King Magog robs four quarters of the world—
E'en now, upon the breadth of all the Earth,
With numbers as the sands upon the sea—
Satan at head, comes forth to desolate;
The Camp of Saints to compass with his hosts
Till Hell and Death shall ghost—City of God!
All things before him down to ruin sink
And hurl'd to desolation all behind:—
Ziona! he brings woes that have not come!
Grim Death and War roar round thee to devour
And Desolation groaneth to receive.

'Three years have roll'd their nothingness to graves

Since Gog, true servant of the Evil one
Came forth to battle with the sons of Light,
And give their brow the holy martyr's crown:
This wall still bids defiance to his hosts,
Stands firm as first—Ziona's tower of strength—
One thousand miles of wall strong as a world!
The City heeds the warring Nations not,
But all her avocations she pursues
And walks with Duty as in days of peace—
Right onward in the busy walks of life
And valiant ever for the cause of Christ.
O, Temperance! thou true Jerusalem-blade!
Thou chaseth Poverty, Sin, Death, Disease—
One half the woes of Earth thy presence fly!
Thou, Ediona's Angel art and guide,
And who shall harm of all the hosts of Hell?
Wo, Famine, Pestilence flee from her gates
And her life's close is but time's slow decay,
While beastly and self-murderous hosts of Gog
By thousands rush to Hell before their time
And drunkards graves hide Gluttony and Lust
Of all his hosts, ten thousand 'lone remain,
Yet stands the wall and Ediona lives.

'I 've not yet supp'd with thee loved one of
Heaven!
Wo lingers not, and Indignation 's near:
Death 's on thy walls and Ruin at thy gates—
When Mercy's smile forsakes, Hell's wrath devours.
Thy tears and carnage, agonies and groans
Shall music be and a right-royal feast.
Fire, sword and Consternation and Dismay
With Rage shall up in arms and shake the world.
Eternal Ruin, Devastation—wake!
Wake Vengeance! walk Creation as in Hell,
While Grim Death makes Existence all his own
And stamps his name on heart of all save Heaven.

'Midnight! Eternity-rob'd and world-ey'd!
Art thou and Heaven a-search for heart-secrets
Lock'd deeply in breast-darkness of mankind?
Search me—Night! ope my bosom's lowest deep
And scan my soul's wide hell and 'twill blast thee!
I am of every mortal thing the curse—
One curse—eternal and almighty all—
Beginning of all horrors and the end!
Thou sleep-eyed Night! thy poppies blossom round,

But thy Lethean fount flies from Death's lip
While men sleep and forget that they are worms.
Ziona sleeps! upon her pillow—Heaven!
Her conscience pure, reflecting—peace of God,
While Seraphs romp and mingle with her dreams!
Awake—arise! ye shall weep blood for this,—
Behold, I am your flood and flame of fire,
And with my rage who 's able to contend?
Thy couch of down shall be thy bed of death,
Bosom's serene the home of fell Despair.
Come Scythe! thou drankest blood of first man slain—
When will thy hunger gorge upon the last?

'The Dragon seats himself on Earth's wide lap—
E'en in Ziona's heart him I behold!
Then hath Hell come to man on this side death.
On his night-frown grim Vengeance hangs with
fiends;
Flame-eyes roll lightning-looks that smite with bolts;
His soul sulphurous burns an Erebus—
He seems like Pit Infernal seen afar!
Hell grows outrageous as a sea for prey:—
The war of Armageddon hath commenc'd,

And Desolation's horrors are at hand!
I will descend, and woo and win and wed
This Bride of God—divine Ziona mine,
And aid Apolyon and his mighty host
To light the Virgin to the bed of Death.'

'He comes—he comes! With his vast Army comes—
Magog, and all the heroes under Heaven!'
A thousand voices cry with wild uproar.
Sleep-lock'd pavilions burst them into life
And pour their warriors forth—flooding the Isle.
Dust-clouds thick-rolling darken all the heavens;
A million torches chase the frown of night,
While Gog beholds their coming and is glad,—
Sees Earth a-swarm with life, and bright in arms
A world-wide Army dreadful to the sight!
Hears clang of arms loud rattling from the rocks,
The sound of wild steed's foot smiting the plain,
And his full soul grows in his bosom's tower.
Wild boars, with anger bristle and affright,
While wolves snuff air and fly to dens afar.
Army to Army joyous greetings shout,—

Not louder speaks Niagara, when quakes
Wide shores around and all the caverns groan.
Like Ocean's countless waves they pour along
Their numbers without number infinite.
Fierce-sweeping cars dash stormy o'er the field;
War-steeds loud neigh—like tempests bounding on;
Hoarse bugles scream; air-rending trumpets shriek,
And pealing drums roll thunderings up to heaven.
Loud roars their coming! Echo, from her home
Of adamant, speeds bellowing up the skies:—
Commotion vast and noise and tumult are
Beyond the mad Atlantic's boisterous roar
When Heaven comes down with world-consuming
rage
And rides her Tempest-steed league-bounding on
O'er cloud-contending heroes of his breast.

Ziona sprang from couch e'er full awake,
And statue-like stood stiff'ning with alarm—
Confounded, terror-rooted to her place!
A thousand heroes leap'd upon her wall—
Gaz'd—still'd with horror mute and dumb amaze,
Till bell of state aloud to council called.

The Senate pour'd flooding the Capital;
Down sat impatient, wary and confus'd.
When fill'd seats spake—'Assembly all conven'd,'
The ripe in wisdom and the full of days—
MAGI! chief, father of his people rose
With loved Ziona bleeding in his heart
And Wisdom's glories daying him around
By chair of state he stood the council's light—
White in his locks and honor'd like a god!
He look'd a prayer to Heaven, then spake aloud
To know that Ediona's hope was God
And her great soul-heroic—Valor's fire.

'Sons, senators and servants of the Highest!
The world 's before us—Ediona's foe!
How can Ziona stand to Earth opposed?
How answer when all Nations smite her gates?
Trust ye your safety to your granite wall?
It cannot stand against an Earth-wide foe,—
It is at best a short respite from Doom.
Destruction is about us as the wind,—
Devourous Ruin bellows in our ears.
Behold! are we a feather on the storm?

Look to the foe! How terrible their power!
The hills are burthen'd with the mighty hosts;
Rocks split asunder 'neath their dreadful load,
And the deep-seated vales, afar shaken!
Fell Devastation widens out their paths;
Before them, all things vanish like a mist,
And hurl'd to desolation all behind:—
Ziona is a very little thing!
Count ye the stars of night, and number them;—
Ah! who can battle with infinitude?
Let thousands fall, and still they seem the same,—
Ten thousand more, and yet we miss them not,
Then thrice ten thousand add! The mighty hosts
Flooding the plain remain invulnerable,
And who shall dare oppose their might save Heaven?
With their broad bucklers wall'd on all sides round
To clashing swords impenetrable stand
Dealing out death in sport to whom they will—
Aplay with heroes as we play with toys!
From Earth's poles, conquering, but not conquer'd
come;
They come to lay God's city desolate:—
Shall Ediona fall! Council decide.'

He said, and down upon the chair of state
With gold and gems and ivory bright, sat mute;
Impatient most to hear his Country's voice
Roll trumpet-toned from every hero's lip—
'*Fear not the frightful coming of the foe.*'
HEROKA, rose, with dignity and grace;
King-majesty sat on his brow with ease;
The mild of soul, the pious, noble, brave—
Forever found in Virtue's path of peace,
And his life's day was one straight march to God.
The big, round tear swell'd in his manly eye,
While thus full soul flow'd out in eloquence:

'Ye wisdom-lights and guides of Ediona!
The storm of peril spreads to huge extent,
And every moment now grows big with death.
Is Piety then mark'd with seal of Fate,
And Mercy's smile clean gone forever-more?
Doth Virtue's end draw near? And will she rest
In solemn quiet of an earthly tomb?
Must sacred Ediona sleep in dust,
And the Almighty own no church below?
Is not Ziona chosen of the Lord?

Then shall she stand—confounded never-more!
'Tis Sin, not Virtue, God casts down to hell,—
He 's on our side! Can Magog war with Him?
The conquest with the Lord of Battles is.
To Sin, our God is a consuming fire—
He frowns forever on his enemies,
But he will crown his chosen people still.

'Our wall 's too weak to hold the Dragon out;
Then let us forth to battle on the plain—
For dreadful battle seems the will of Heaven.
The Lord helps those alone who help themselves,—
If we sow not, no harvests may we reap;
If Ediona will not smite her foe
Her brow cannot be crown'd with victory,
But Idleness shall perish in her rags,
And Sluggishness to his long death go down:
Heaven calls alike on all to do our part
And trust to God for conquest at His hand.
The cause of Justice draws the sword—help Heaven!
In self-defence we war—we fight for Peace
For Innocence and Virtue ever fair,—
Religion, Freedom battle on our side,

And they shall be to us the power of God
In hurling forth of fell Iniquity!
O! let us rise with full of faith in God
Our light of hope and our great victory.'

He ceas'd, and sighed in spirit as he sat.
GODOWNI, then, in princely grandeur rose,
Whose sage-like look spake hero and a saint,
And Wisdom's home and Council's depth re-
veal'd:—
A God-like hero from his early youth,
And the most manly man of men alive,—
The head and hand of War—the Victory!
Attention mute hung breathless o'er the hall
While Eloquence rode forth as voice of Heaven,
And thus aloud spake thunderings of his soul
Till all hearts fill'd with manna from on high:

'Count not our foe ye chosen of the Lord!
Say, who are Magog's hosts compar'd with ours?
A drunken rabble, cowards, villains, slaves
Drove by Oppression's lash and Tyranny
Against their will to battle at our gates,

And led by Dragon—captive at his will.
They number cowards when they count their droves,
We, number heroes where we number men,
While God of battles is our strength and tower.
True valor makes our numbers numberless—
Say, who shall count the army of the Lord?
His chosen few are more than seashore's sand,
And stars of night are not God-bless'd as they:
God's Ediona—world of heroes is!
She 's Bravery's self—a hero God-ordain'd;
Her little armies countless thousands are—
A number without number—infinite!
Strong Valor's might is like the wind of heaven—
What scales can weigh, what tongue can tell its
power?
'Tis a divinity—Ziona's crown.
Can weakness be when every arm 's a host?
Nations our strength, heroes our people are
And God of Armies our defence for aye.
When he is for us who can be against?
Can Magog's millions then compare with us?
They are but dust upon the winds of Heaven,—
Them, God shall sweep to ruin in his wrath

And smile upon his people and deliver.
He falleth on his foes and who can hinder?
Roll'd not the Red Sea back for Israel's sake
And give their Egypt-foe to watery graves?
The Lord our God 's Omnipotent to save,
But where he frowns there is Oblivion.
Why doubt we then? Where is discouragement?
To disbelieve, is an offence to Him—
To trust in God, the wisdom of the Bless'd.

'Who number us the oaks on Oren's Hills,
Or count the leaves that fan the summer hours?
Storm comes, and leaves and forests are no more!
How countless too are Ocean's mountain-waves?
Yet Tempest drives before him in his ire
And hurls them all to ruin with a breath!
Those legions shadow vale and hill afar,
As numberless as dews our enemy—
An earth-wide army and a world of men!
But who shall face Heaven's heroes in the field?
Who stand when Ediona meets her foe?
Her rising up in arms is terrible;
Her march to field is Tempest in his rage;

Her might in battle smites as bolts of God;
Deaths from her hand like fires from Etna leap,
While Fury heaps her death-path down to Hell:
Who but the Dragon then will think of flight?
Darkness shall flee the rising up of day,
And Satan fall like lightning—thundersmote!
Peace, liberty are with the Lord our God,
And he will crown his Ediona still.
War is our safety and our God our hope—
Our sword unsheathed shall set Ziona free.
I charge thee Ediona—rise! to arms!
Go forth in God, and laurel'd Victory
Asmile, shall wave her star-gem'd flag to thee.'

Thus spake he loud, and ended thus, and sat.
KILLMORI, rose, the swift of foot and bold
In fight—the tempest and the bolt of war—
A battle-driving spirit consummate!
In polished arms, and spread a living light
O'er listning heroes thronging him around.
His face of cloud, portentious spake of storm,—
War-kindling eye talk'd with soul of fire
While thus the troubled Council he address'd:

'Ye lights in peace and thunderbolts in storm!
Our strength hath slumber'd long and quietly,
But Danger's cry wakes up the hero's soul.
Our country's safety calls us to the field;
That voice is sacred—oracle of God.
King Magog's every-nation'd army comes,—
Red battle 's 'fore us with its field of blood,
And War loud roars at Valor to awake!
Earth, Heaven and Hell demand the sacrifice:
Death's all devouring hunger must be gorged
By wasteful vengeance and the fiery sword.
Ye senators and heroes world-renown'd!
Doth coming tempest darken all our sky?
There 's sunshine, calm and Heaven beyond the
cloud—
Let Valor, Wisdom, Virtue press along.

'The brow of Victory 's crown'd by Heroism
And Bravery battling with the world, conquers.
Doth the intrepid lion e'er regard
A million emmets trailing cross his path,
Or heed ten thousand gnats perch'd on his mane?
Behold! our lovely island stands secure

Amid a sea of waves, and one firm rock
Defies the mighty Ocean's dreadful rush,—
Yon hill 's unmoved by all the storms of time!
Rock and hill-like we planted are by God
Himself—fast as foundation of the globe;
Then who can harm the chosen bride of God?
Yon Dragon-host?—a bacchanalian mob!
They will away as dust before the storm—
One hero can a thousand cowards chase,
Yea, two of us may put them all to flight!
Could Magog number slaves as forests boughs,
Or wilderness both trees and leaves, and shade
Creation with the billions infinite,
Ziona would not fear—she is of God!
Pale fear within her sacred walls lives not,—
When Dragon drove our fathers to this isle
Fear was excluded quite; they knew but this:
To bravely live and how to bravely die.

'Ziona is the land of valor still
The home of heroes—nursery of the brave,
And she shall still be Freedom's own beloved
Or martyr's holy tomb forever-more.

Our country 's sacred next to God and Heaven;
For this loved isle we dare contend with Death,
And we will leave her only for our graves;
While there is life, our bosoms are her shield—
Long as we stand, we 'll stand 'twixt her and doom:—
Then let death come—he 'll find us at our posts.
All those who die shall wear the hero's crown,
And they will fall a sacrifice to God:
At Duty's side we fall if fall we must,
And there stand heroes till we sink in death.
We can die veterans,—servants shall we live—
Base slaves to Dragon and Tartarean hosts?
We 've lived with God and learn'd his love by heart;
We know not how, nor will we ever learn
To serve Pollution and Iniquity!
We 've lived with glory—with renown we 'll die,—
We scorn to outlive virtue and our fame—
Death and the grave, not life and infamy!
For Liberty and Right our all we stake—
Our life for Freedom shall be freely given.
The blood of heroes glorifies the field,
And Valor sunk to rest sleeps quietly.

'My soul is war—sword flames to meet the foe!
There 's nothing left but arms and hope in God—
Us, on they 'll lead to glorious victory.
Our host must meet their hosts, our sword their
swords:
If war we must, why longer here debate!
In fight immediate the triumph lies,
And danger, ruin, death in slow delay.
Our foes to night hold joyous festival
With dance and song and bacchanalian glee;
Shall we at waking up of rosy Dawn
One gall-drop add to their full cup of bliss,
And let them feel the terror of our arms?
Are we the laugh of enemies to night,
And shall we not their groan tomorrow be?
Then face them bravely as becomes the brave.
Our country now loud calls her heroes forth,—
She calls upon her sons in her great need;
Will they not stand unshaken at her side
And save their mother from the Dragon's jaws?
To shrink from duty seals Ziona's fate:
Then let us march with confidence in God,
And hope shall ripen into victory.'

'We 'll stake our lives and fortunes for her sake,'
A thousand voices cried with loud acclaim,
'And march with her to victory or death;
Yea, we will battle with our Dragon-foe
Tho' Ruin be around him as a storm
And Devastation desolates his path!
Count not but show to us the enemy,—
Lead thou, Godowni! Heaven-anointed chief—
Thou victory-gaining hero of renown!
Ziona hails thee generalissimo.
To arms—to arms! Ziona shall be free.'

The people thus with tearful energy
Spake out their souls with holy ardor fired
Brightning for dreadful battle all around,
Till father Magi, loved by every heart—
Light of the senate and their wisdom's crown
Arose, and shook the honors of his head,
And order was and silence thro' the hall,
When thus, aloud, his people he address'd:

'Sons! Valor's self lives in your souls of fire!
'Tis joy to see your hearts and country one;

That love is noble—cherish still the flame—
Heaven will reward your zeal with victory.
Elect! from every country under Heaven—
Sons worthy of your sires—go, Virtue-arm'd!
Face peril bravely as becomes the brave,
And trust to God our sacred Liberty,—
Yea, trust in Him and be confounded never.
Successful war ye wage if Heaven but smile,
And victory 's yours if ye to selves prove true.

'Why waste the night in further counsel now
When every hero's voice is loud for war?
Valor's full bosom burns to meet the foe,
And each soul leaps to mingle with the fight,—
No fear in walls of Ediona lives,
For Virtue's eye e'er looks on Victory.
Who save the foe shall tremble when we rise
And Ediona thunders to the field?
Her going forth is like Tornado's rush,—
Vengeance in midst bares his red arm of hell;
Her every sword a very Legion is,
Her arrow's flight the coming-on of Death,
And path's wide-waste a desolation all!

Then let the Army of the Lord arise,
And Magog's sable bands shall melt away
As ghosts of night from world-rejoicing Morn,
Or vapors dank the rising up of Day.
The enemies of God revel and dance
Till Drunkenness and Sleep pile all the plain,—
Up heroes! meet yon Bacchanalian-mob—
Be swords to fight the Battle of the Lord!
Doth Ediona stand on edge of doom?
Let all her warriors now as one brave man
Rush forth, and save her from Oblivion.'

Does the World want the other Six Books?

Princeton, Butler county, Ohio.

www.ingramcontent.com/pod-product-compliance
Lightning Source LLC
LaVergne TN
LVHW010211110826
845151LV00004B/1053

* 9 7 8 1 4 2 5 5 2 8 3 7 9 *